About the author

Caroline Shreeve was born in Huntingdon in 1943 and qualified as a doctor at St Mary's Hospital, Paddington. She then practised as a hospital doctor and as a GP in Britain and in South Africa, later turning her knowledge to the pursuit of medical journalism. Following a symposium on evening primrose oil in 1981 she became interested in the application of herbal medicine. She also trained with the National Council of Psychotherapists as a hypnotherapist.

In her work as physician and hypnotherapist she has specialized in women's emotional problems and is therefore uniquely qualified to tackle the subject of the menopause. In addition to her London degree she is a Fellow of the Royal Society of Medicine and a licentiate of the Royal College of Physicians. She is also a contributor to a number of periodicals which include *Over 21*, *Company* and *She* magazine.

D1387506

Overcoming the Menopause Naturally

Dr Caroline M. Shreeve, MB, BS(London)

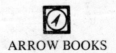

ARROW BOOKS

Arrow Books Limited
62–65 Chandos Place, London WC2N 4NW

An imprint of Century Hutchinson Ltd

London Melbourne Sydney Auckland
Johannesburg and agencies throughout
the world

First published 1986
Century Arrow edition 1986
Reprinted 1987
Arrow edition 1987

Diagram drawn by Joy Fitzsimmons

Photoset by Rowland Phototypesetting Ltd,
Bury St Edmunds, Suffolk

Printed and bound in Great Britain by
Anchor Brendon Ltd, Tiptree, Essex

ISBN 0 09 946680 5

Dedication

This book is dedicated to Barbara Levy in grateful acknowledgement of her advice and encouragement.

Contents

Introduction

The menopause – in our society, at least – has a most unattractive image. It is a time when complex hormonal changes take place, marking the end of a woman's reproductive years and – so far as many women believe – the end of physical attractiveness, sexual enjoyment, and the illusion of 'still being young'.

Of course, some women in their forties or fifties – especially those who suffer from difficult periods or find contraception a nuisance – will say with feeling that they cannot wait for the menopause to relieve them of their problems. Nevertheless, very few women genuinely look forward to losing their fertility, or to entering a phase of their life which indisputably marks the encroachment of the ageing process.

The realization of fertility loss can, in fact, cause more secret grief than many of us would dream of admitting. True, only a small minority of women choose to have babies after the age of forty, and many would find an unexpected pregnancy at this time catastrophic. But there is all the difference in the world between deciding not to conceive, and having the freedom to make that decision taken away from you.

Many women's sexual self-confidence stays happily intact all the time they remain fertile, only to suffer a shattering blow when they enter the menopause. They admit – at least to their friends, and often to their doctors – that they feel they are 'no longer real women' since they can no longer have babies, and that their lives as sexual human beings are at an end.

Part of this reaction results from the effect of hormonal changes upon the mind and emotions; but knowing this is little consolation for suddenly feeling sexless and old. Many women have told me that all the time they were having periods, they felt sexually 'on a par' with most younger women, and sufficiently self-confident to flirt when they felt inclined, 'compete' for younger men, and even contemplate affairs should the occasion arise.

Once their periods stopped, though, they felt a 'Cinderella at midnight' change come over them, as though they had turned into old hags at the chime of a biological clock. They no longer bothered with the sexual sides of their natures. Instead of enjoying their husband's or boyfriend's company, they found themselves bad-tempered, tearful, and frigid, opting for a night at home with a box of chocolates and the television in preference to venturing out into public places where the mere sight of attractive (fertile) younger women would set off an inner turmoil of jealous resentment.

If this reaction to the menopause sounds melodramatic and far-fetched, try to remember how you felt when your periods *started*. Most of us nowadays realize that the menarche (first period) can be an emotionally charged experience for many girls – and that was even more true twenty or thirty years ago when all the preparation many of us got for menstruation was a school biology lesson on the reproductive habits of the rabbit, or a whispered – mostly inaccurate – account of what to expect from a school chum.

Times have changed very much for the better with respect to our attitudes to the facts of life. Some of us would add that they have gone too far, with an overemphasized liberality on sexual matters resulting in widespread promiscuity at a young age. That may be so, yet it remains a fact that knowledge and understanding are a great deal healthier than ignorance and fear, and that women throughout their reproductive lives profit in one way or another from the lifting of the veil from old taboo subjects.

Periods have acquired a far more acceptable image than they at one time had. Advertisements appear throughout the women's press, on the Underground and even on the sides of buses, for prettily packaged slim sanitary towels, as well as for internal tampons, and the menarche is used as the advertising theme for one of the towel brands, in which it is hailed as the (presumably desirable) change from 'little girl to woman'.

Painful periods, too, are discussed at length, in magazine articles, on radio and TV, and in schools and at work. Most women realize that they no longer have to tolerate severe menstrual pain or PMS, and know what to buy over the counter or to ask for on prescription should the problem arise. Sexual difficulties, impotence, frigidity, preference for one's own sex, and unusual sexual practices have all come out into the open forum of free discussion; even incest has been used as part of the theme of a recent best-seller.

Is the same happy fate likely to befall the menopause? Will 'the change' ever be an event women will be encouraged to look forward to, as marking a new, exciting development in their lives? Will it one day be given a good press, and the bogeymen notions of hot flushes, an expanding girth and painful intercourse, dismissed?

None of this seems likely at the moment. In the public's mind, the menopause and mothers-in-law have a good deal in common; both are inherently nasty, better not thought about, and most effectively dealt with by cracking music hall jokes about them. And there is a fundamental reason why this concept is unlikely to change. The menopause – at present, at any rate – offers pharmaceutical and surgical product companies little commercial opportunity on the open market compared with the specially formulated pain killers, wide variety of sanitary protection, and herbal remedies known to be useful for menstrual problems.

How much of the underlying fear about the menopause is warranted? Certainly if one turns to nature for guidance, her rhythmic cycles are based impartially upon the age-old theme of birth, life and death, and we can see, in the life cycles of the natural world, as much beauty in the fallen rose petal, the hag moon and the burnt ochre of autumn, as we can in the germinating seed, the virgin moon and the brilliant greens of spring.

Whether or not you feel that to be natural we should give up trying to clutch at a disappearing youthfulness and grow old gracefully, depends upon your individual point of view. But since the 'change of life' can come at the early age of forty (it can arrive earlier, but is then defined as 'premature'), and since female life expectancy has increased remarkably since 1900 from approximately 50 to 82 years, any woman can expect to spend one third of her life or longer as post-menopausal (1).

Another fact that follows from our greatly extended life expectancy, is that the age range of 'old' age has altered. When death might reasonably be expected to occur between the ages of fifty and sixty, women were considerably older at, say, the age of forty-five than is the case nowadays, although admittedly disease and malnutrition were a more frequent cause of death at that time than the ageing process itself.

There seems to me every reason why women in their forties, fifties, and older should make every effort to retain their youthfulness. Far from 'flying in the face of nature' as one forty-five year-old menopausal patient remarked to me resentfully, making use of all that a natural diet, natural supplements, natural beauty products and – where necessary – natural medicine have to offer, is the safest, surest way of allowing ourselves – physically and mentally – to achieve our highest potential.

Few botanists, geneticists and biochemists are criticized for unnatural activities when they use modern technology and science to breed healthier and more productive plants and animals than have evolved under natural conditions. Likewise, there is no reason for us to feel embarrassed or ashamed if we use every natural device at our disposal to keep healthy, attractive and fulfilled.

How, then, should we regard the menopause? As a natural step in our development to physical, mental and spiritual maturity, and most emphatically not as a ghastly if inevitable experience through which all normal women are obliged to pass on the way to the grave. The menopause is no more a disorder than are monthly periods or the menarche, and should produce no symptoms that cannot be swiftly and effectively dealt with by natural means.

If this sounds thoroughly unrealistic, in view of all your mother, friends and relations have told you about the 'change', or of your own experiences of hot flushes, night sweats, palpitations, joint pains and depression, let me assure you that simple, practical help is at hand. Here is a regimen designed to help your menopause pass with minimum discomfort, and to put you on the road to better health and happiness than you have ever enjoyed before, without the use of artificial hormones.

One word of caution. Following a daily regimen that requires a number of lifestyle changes, demands self-discipline, and this presents even more of a challenge when you are required to alter a longstanding attitude to this phase of your life. Don't be tempted to rush things and make all the necessary changes instantly.

Adopt different aspects of the programme one at a time, and be patient – and your progress will be far greater than if you adopted the crash-dieter's approach. Attempting to rectify years of over-weight – or in this case, a less than perfect lifestyle – in a couple of weeks is destined to fail.

The following chapters set out firstly to explain what happens to the female body during and after menopause; secondly, to sketch out the lifestyle plan which is the basic purpose of this book; and thirdly, to look at the various forms of natural remedies that are available to every woman wishing to make use of them.

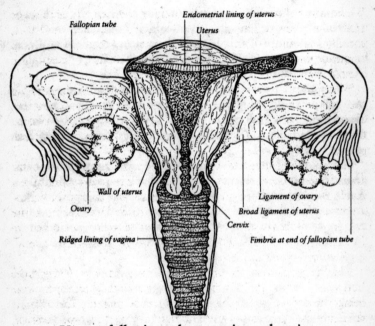

Fallopian tube

Endometrial lining of uterus

Uterus

Ligament of ovary

Wall of uterus

Broad ligament of uterus

Ovary

Cervix

Ridged lining of vagina

Fimbria at end of fallopian tube

Uterus, fallopian tubes, ovaries and vagina

Chapter One

Why the menopause happens

We commonly use the word 'menopause' to mean all the changes that take place at the end of a woman's reproductive phase, usually spanning a period of between two and three years. I shall continue to use the word in this way, but in fact its real meaning is simply the 'last menstrual period'.

The medical term for what we generally call the menopause, is the 'climacteric'. The final menstrual bleed occurs during the climacteric, which in turn is defined medically as 'the two to three year transitional period during which reproductive function ceases' (1).

No one is still quite sure why the menopause happens at all. But to understand what we do know about it, it is necessary to take a quick look at the events occurring each month during the reproductive years. The regularity of the menstrual cycle is due to the regularity with which ovulation takes place, that is, the release from the ovary of a mature ovum, or egg, contained within a small hollow, the ovarian follicle.

This happens once about every twenty-eight days, somewhere between day ten and day fifteen of the monthly cycle (day one being the day on which the previous period began). The ovum is shed into the open end of the fallopian tube of the womb (uterus), into which it is directed by finger-like tentacles, the fimbria. It then starts its journey down the fallopian tube towards the hollow body of the uterus, and the empty ovarian follicle in the ovary develops into a tiny gland, the corpus luteum (the 'yellow body').

These events in the cycle are governed by two hormones

produced by the master endocrine gland – the pituitary – within the brain, in turn regulated by the control centre of the menstrual cycle within the hypothalamus. This is an area of specialized brain tissue about the size of a greengage and situated immediately above the pituitary gland in the floor of the front part of the brain.

The first of these two hormones, FSH (follicle stimulating hormone), stimulates the ovum to ripen and to produce oestrogen. This hormone reconstitutes the lining of the uterus which has been depleted by the previous menstrual bleed, thus preparing it to receive a fertilized ovum, should fertilization take place.

The second of the pituitary hormones, LH (luteinizing hormone), starts to be secreted instead of FSH once the ovum has burst out of the ovary and reached the fallopian tube. It is responsible for the development of the corpus luteum, which now secretes progesterone and only a small amount of oestrogen. These cause further changes in the endometrium (lining of the uterus), including further thickening and an increase in its blood supply. If the ripe ovum travels the length of its fallopian tube without meeting a sperm and it reaches the interior of the uterus without becoming fertilized, it shrivels up and is discarded with the next menstrual loss. The production of progesterone by the corpus luteum starts to diminish around day twenty-two. When the blood level of progesterone has fallen to a certain level, the lining of the uterus is shed as menstrual blood, beginning on average around day twenty-eight (the next cycle's day one).

(Should the ovum meet sperm in the fallopian tube and become fertilized, it travels down the tube into the uterus where it embeds itself in the lining of the wall and starts to develop into an embryo. In this case, instead of shrivelling up, the corpus luteum secretes hormones essential to pregnancy.)

The ripe follicles in each of the two ovaries develop from future ova which start off life among the germinal cells in the outer surface covering of the ovaries. This occurs before the girl baby is born, and during the first six months of life. Future ova bore downwards into the tissue of the ovary, where each forms a primitive (primordial) follicle enveloped in membrane. Only a small percentage of the total number of primordial follicles finally develops into mature ovarian follicles.

The ovary has a second very important function to perform, besides the production of ova. It manufactures and secretes oestrogen, responsible for the complete development of female sexual characteristics. This endocrine activity is also under the control of the pituitary gland.

Since no ova are produced, and no primordial follicles formed after the age of six months, the supply is depleted slightly every time ovulation occurs. As the total number of ova becomes exhausted, oestrogen production declines despite continued secretion of FSH by the pituitary. The falling level of oestrogen in the blood – in particular, of the type known as 'oestradiol' made only by the ovary – is the most important cause of menopausal symptoms.

Finally the ovaries shrink, and within four to five years after the last period, the last few follicles disappear and the ovaries consist only of the connective tissue framework (stroma) in which the follicles were once found.

Although the ovaries no longer secrete oestrogen, other varieties of this hormone – chiefly oestrone – continue to be synthesized, mainly from androgens (male sex hormones) produced by the ovaries and the adrenal glands. (Women manufacture a small quantity of male sex hormones throughout their reproductive years, and boys and men synthesize small quantities of female hormones as well.)

This oestrogen synthesis takes place for the most part in the fat layers beneath the skin. To a certain extent, the oestrone made in this way compensates for the deficiency of ovarian-produced oestradiol. If you are overweight, then you make more oestrone than if you are thin, and as a result may very well suffer less severely from menopausal symptoms than you would if your body weight were normal. However, this in no way provides a good excuse for not slimming!

The average age at which women have their last menstrual period in this country is 51.4 years. There are three main ways in which it is likely to happen. Firstly, your periods may just stop. You may have a normal period one month, never suspecting it to be your last – which it may turn out to be.

Secondly, the intervals between your periods may gradually get longer and longer, until eventually they fade out altogether. Thirdly, the amount of blood you lose each month can slowly grow less and less until you finally lose none at all.

It is well worth emphasizing here that post-menopausal bleeding (i.e. bleeding occurring a year or more after your periods have stopped) is never normal. Thorough investigation of this important symptom involves a D and C (dilation and curettage, or womb scrape), and you should never be persuaded to agree to less than this.

The Advantages

Let's look briefly at the advantages to be gained from reaching the menopause. There definitely *are* several points to be made in its favour, and you don't have to 'scrape the bottom of the barrel' to find them, either.

CONTRACEPTION
Firstly, there is no further need for contraception (but see below). This may not affect you one way or the other, if you are unattached, or have relied for years upon a form of contraception which has given you no trouble. For many women, though, the menopause means the end of an IUCD (intra-uterine contraceptive device), monthly courses of micro-dose contraceptive pills, or the cap, diaphragm or sponge, all of which cause problems to a number of users.

IUCDs are relatively trouble-free, but capable of producing severe menstrual pain and very heavy bleeding in a number of women – many of whom put up with the undesirable side effects because of the device's other advantages. The mini-Pill specially designed for older women contains – of course – as low a dose of sex hormones as are safely compatible with a reliable contraceptive effect. All the same, nothing can eliminate totally the slight risk of cancer and thrombosis, even though this has been reduced to an absolute minimum.

By contrast, the cap or diaphragm – usually used in conjunction with a spermicidal cream – is relatively free of side effects. But this method is unarguably fiddly, messy and difficult to combine with the type of spontaneous love-making many couples enjoy, since it necessitates several minutes of preparation in the bathroom beforehand.

Besides the methods already mentioned, many couples are equally relieved when they no longer have to rely upon the male sheath, the rhythm method or coitus interruptus as a means of contraception. The rhythm method can be unreliable unless several factors denoting the time of fertility are taken carefully into account.

Coitus interruptus (the man withdrawing before ejaculation, and climaxing outside his partner's body) is used by some couples who claim that they find it trouble-free. Nevertheless, it is known to be unreliable since sperm can be present in the fluid secreted from the penis before ejaculation occurs. It is also considered to be psychologically and emotionally stressful, with neither partner deriving full satisfaction from their love-making.

The sheath is reliable but can be a nuisance to remember, and some men object to it on the grounds that it diminishes the sensitivity of the penis during intercourse. Any vaginal soreness or dryness in the woman is also likely to be aggravated by the use of a rubber condom.

It is also worth mentioning that all the above methods of birth control with the exception of the IUCD, coitus interruptus and the rhythm method are possible causes of recurrent attacks of cystitis and urethritis. Some women who suffer from chronic urinary problems find that they are no longer troubled once they stop using the cap, spermicidal cream or the Pill.

However you may feel about no longer having to use contraceptives, though, don't be tempted to stop all precautions just because you *think* your periods have stopped. It is still possible to conceive up to one year after the last menstrual bleed, and to be on the safe side I prefer to advise women to continue with their normal method of birth control for eighteen months after their last period.

This may seem like erring unnecessarily on the side of caution, but you will probably agree that an unwanted pregnancy – or an abortion – are the very last things you feel like facing just at the moment.

PERIOD PAINS/PMS

Other advantages of the menopause include freedom from possibly painful, heavy and inconvenient periods, and from the premenstrual syndrome (PMS). Period pains and accompanying symptoms (headaches, nausea, faintness) tend to get better as time goes by, being especially severe in teenagers and women in their twenties, and often disappearing with the birth of the first baby. They can, however, continue right up to the time of the menopause, and cause considerable problems every month by interfering with work, home and social life. They may also need painkillers and other drugs before relief is experienced, and these in turn can cause side effects.

PMS, on the other hand, is more likely to be present at the time of the menopause because in contrast to period problems, it has a tendency to grow more severe as the years pass. Premenstrual symptoms can be as troublesome – if not more so – than menstrual problems, especially the psychological ones of irritability and temper outbursts. PMS and its attendant depression quite often make women feel extremely pessimistic – both about their present symptoms and their future menopause.

There are of course natural remedies both for PMS and for dysmenorrhoea (difficult periods), but few GPs are aware of the efficacy of many of them. Consequently, thousands of prescriptions are written monthly for analgesics, the contraceptive Pill and prostaglandin inhibitors (for period problems), and for diuretics (water pills), pain-killers, tranquillizers and anti-depressants for PMS.

SEXUAL ACTIVITY

There are as many different attitudes to sex during and after the menopause, as there are menopausal and post-menopausal women to have them. Despite the myriad individual variations, though, here are four pretty typical ones chosen from the case notes of menopausal clinic patients:

1 Mrs T. R., aged 51: 'It is not "nice" to indulge in sex once you reach (say) the age of fifty; as for "it" taking place between senior citizens – it's positively obscene!'

2 Mrs M. B., aged 48: 'Sex has always been a bore and a nuisance – now I can claim vaginal soreness as an excuse, and hopefully after six months to a year of abstinence, he'll forget all about it . . .'

3 Mrs J. S., aged 42: 'I am fat and ugly, it'll probably hurt, I'm tired and headachy and I don't feel like it; anyway, I couldn't bear him to see me without any clothes on, my figure's so repulsive.'

4 Mrs E. O., aged 46: 'It's marvellous and always has been, and I am sure it is going to get better and better – if that's possible – since we won't even have to stop for my periods!'

Not many revelations about sexual attitudes are totally frank – either those confided to doctors or those shared between best friends. If our innermost thoughts and fears were that easy to voice, there would be far less need for counselling and psychotherapy, and far fewer prescriptions written annually for anti-depressants and tranquillizers. So it is worth glancing at each of the four opinions given above, to see what they hide about the women concerned.

1 Mrs T. R. never really enjoyed sex. Sex was not really 'nice' even when she first married in her early twenties, and the

responsibility for this lies chiefly with the ultra-strict upbringing she received at home and in Catholic boarding school.

Sex has always seemed 'dirty' to Mrs T. R., and having reached her fifties, she feels that she can at last be free of the obligation. Her rigid moral code of sex being 'for the procreation of children only', though, has never given her any happiness, and she has suffered for a number of years from insomnia, a compulsive hand-washing habit and depression. She is unaware of having missed a great deal that life has to offer, but feels very bitter in a non-specific way.

2 Mrs M. B. doesn't hold strong religious views on sexual activity – she has simply never enjoyed it. This is not the fault of an over-strict upbringing. It is due to the fact that she and her husband married when they were both eighteen, knowing only the bare facts of life, and that they were too shy to discuss 'it' in terms of mutual enjoyment.

Sex has always been the same for them – once a week on Saturday night, in the missionary position, with no questions asked and no requests, or suggestions of varying the technique. She has always given her husband what she regards as his 'marital rights', but hopes that she will not have to continue to do so for much longer.

3 Mrs J. S., on the other hand, *has* enjoyed sex in the past. She had two or three steady boyfriends before marrying at the age of 29, and she and her husband have had a good sex life, sharing a taste for variety and the ability to receive and give pleasure.

Now premenopausal, though, at the early age of forty-two, Mrs J. S. has become depressed at the thought of the ageing process. She is particularly aware of the two extra stone in weight which have accumulated over the past two years. Lacking in self-confidence, she claims lack of interest instead, but her excuses hide misery and fear, and her suppressed sexual urges express themselves in fits of crying and unaccustomed outbursts of rage.

4 On the surface, Mrs E. O. sounds highly enviable. But without being cynical, there is something slightly manic about her claims of superlative sexual enjoyment. Few women – or men – find sex with the same person for twenty-five years quite so scintillating as she claims to find it. If they do, they are usually the first to admit that, like every other aspect of marriage, sex is a great deal better at certain times than at others, and *can* occasionally prove less than totally fulfilling.

Mrs E. O. does, in fact, have her own share of worry and doubt. A successful model for ten years, and now the part-owner of a well-known model agency, she deals daily with beautiful young girls in their 'teens and early twenties.

She has serious doubts about her own attractions, as she sees the expected signs of ageing in her skin and hair, and worries about whether her husband, who has always been a womanizer, will continue to find her attractive.

Sexual and marital counselling are not usually given unless requested by patients – but quite a large number of women do seek advice from their doctors in this connection during their forties and fifties. It is easy to see how marriages can become severely strained during the menopause. If sex has been simply tolerated, as it was by Mrs T. R., the 'change' is more or less bound to be used as an excuse for finally giving it up.

This particular patient's husband, fortunately, was very sympathetic to his wife's feelings and did not try to coerce her to continue 'relations' with him. But a number of marriages *do* come adrift after twenty-five to thirty years when sex is discontinued – even if it has never been a highly pleasurable experience for either partner.

Mrs M. B.'s marriage nearly ended shortly after our talk during which she told me her feelings about sex. She discovered that her husband was having an affair with a woman at work – some five years her own senior! She was devastated – as was her husband when she told him that she had found out – and they both came to see me together. He by this time had ended his affair – and freely admitted that he had only sought it in the first place for sexual pleasure.

'After all, M. has never really enjoyed it,' he said, and she was honest enough to agree with him. The culmination was that both made a great effort to put their marriage back on secure ground – and they agreed, once they had considered my suggestion, to attend a sexual therapy clinic.

Couples of all ages are seen at these clinics, and M. was willing to find out whether she might yet learn to enjoy sex – encouraged no doubt by her husband's ex-mistress' age! (The therapy was a success.)

Mrs J. S. was probably the least complicated of the four women to advise. She had a loving, tolerant if somewhat bewildered husband who had been very upset by her recent outbursts of temper – and came along with his wife to discuss their marital problems. We discussed some of the doubts she was experiencing, and he was astounded to discover that she considered herself ugly and unappealing.

They went on a diet together, took up cycling, and discussed their sexual feelings honestly. Once J. understood that many of her menopausal problems could be overcome naturally, she began to put the advice into practice, and a year later had regained both her premenopausal figure and her self-confidence.

The case of Mrs E. O. had a less happy outcome. I only saw her at the menopause clinic in the first place because she was suffering from occasional hot flushes – and the subject of sex came up because I enquired whether she experienced any vaginal dryness. She came to see me six months later, suffering from depression – her husband had left her for one of her own models, and she confided in me then how she had worried that she was losing her looks.

The sad, sometimes tragic, side of much of the fear and regret engendered by the menopause, is that there is no need for them. The arrival of the menopause no more signifies the end of your personal development and the beginning of a gradual decline into senility, than your menarche (first period) signified the commencement of your growth and personal development.

You had been maturing, physically and mentally – and your personality had been growing more complex – for some ten to fifteen years before your first period arrived. It signified that you were developing normally, and that your endocrine glands were ready to start off your menstrual cycle. But it was not the only – or even the most important – milestone of your developmental progress.

In exactly the same way, your last period means simply that your ovaries are ceasing to secrete oestrogen. The reproductive phase of your life has come to an end. The implications of this change are, undeniably, enormous. But the menopause is neither a disease nor a catastrophe. It is the end of your 'reproductive phase' – I never use the expression 'your reproductive life' – and the start of a new phase in your personal development.

It is true that, for many of us, having babies is such a totally fulfilling experience that the prospect of no longer being fertile seems intolerable. All the same, there are a number of ways of approaching this issue. It seems sensible to me, if the future without pregnancies looks bleak, to accept that giving birth and rearing a family have been the richest and most rewarding aspects of life to date. But to make quite certain not to write off the future years as useless, just because they are not able to offer the same experience.

Here is the advice I give to less fortunate women who are approaching – or in the middle of – the menopause, and have never been able to have children despite longing for them. Don't refuse to acknowledge your disappointment, since this is the only way to come to terms with it. If you feel especially depressed about it, talk about it to your husband, lover, mother or best friend – or simply write your feelings down in an exercise book, expressing your feelings exactly as they are.

If you are angry, bitter and jealous – instead of storing your feelings as resentment, give vent to them in a constructive way. Write a poem (it doesn't have to be 'good'), smash a tennis or squash ball round a court twice a week, or take up jogging. Whatever you do, refuse to let your disappointment and unhappiness accumulate – this is guaranteed to harm you in the end.

Also remember that the menopause only signifies the end of your fertility. It does *not* mean the end of sexual attractiveness or enjoyment, any more than it means that you are bound to put on weight, lose your hair by the combful, and develop wrinkles and sagging skin overnight. If you go about it the right way, you can retain your youthful good looks for many years to come – and, what is equally important, remain healthy, happy and self-confident.

Many women discover another bonus to approaching the menopause positively. Instead of losing their 'usefulness' to their family, i.e. their sense of identity as 'childbearer-wife-mother', they discover new depths to their relationships with their partner, and their children if they have them.

The saying that 'like begets like' is true. Money seems to come to those who already have it; and success certainly does breed success. The greater your own personal involvement with life and people, the more other people will want to draw you into their lives and share joys and problems with you.

You may well be wondering quite how a positive attitude helps with such problems as hot flushes, night sweats, headaches, irritability, poor memory and concentration, and stiff, aching joints. They are certainly all associated with the menopause – but they are not all related to a falling oestrogen level. There is evidence to suggest that the busier the life you lead, the less likely you are to suffer from them. In addition, we now know for certain that all these symptoms are aggravated by poor diet, insufficient exercise, anxiety and stress factors.

All menopausal symptoms arise basically from a natural, physical process and in most cases respond very well to natural remedies. In the next chapter we will have a look at menopausal symptoms in detail, and at the orthodox approach to treatment, before we consider the natural approach.

Chapter Two

How problems arise

Because of the varying opinions about the advantages and disadvantages of hormone replacement therapy (HRT), menopausal symptoms have been studied by orthodox doctors in great detail. One of the main purposes of the clinical trials has been to distinguish between menopausal symptoms which really result from oestrogen deficiency, and those due to the ageing process and social and domestic problems (2).

A number of hospital trials have confirmed the usefulness of supplemental oestrogen in the treatment of hot flushes, night sweats, a sore, dry vagina and increased frequency in passing water. Nevertheless, HRT is not at all popular with menopausal women, and a report in the *British Medical Journal* in 1984 (3) suggested that fewer than 2% were willing to accept it as a form of treatment. Later in this chapter we will take a look at HRT since, although this book is about overcoming the menopause by natural means, it is preferable for the choice to be an informed one. Many doctors in all good faith urge their menopausal patients to accept supplemental hormones – and the value of 'alternative' methods of handling the symptoms can only be judged fairly when the relative benefits of the two approaches have been examined.

There are two main types of problem associated with the menopause. Firstly, there are the symptoms commonly experienced at that time, such as hot flushes, night sweats, vaginal soreness, irritability and anxiety. These are often known collectively as the 'menopausal syndrome'. Secondly, there are the changes in bone structure that occur, involving pronounced 'thinning' of the bone substance and a reduction in its density, known medically as osteoporosis.

Approximately 70% of all women suffer from the menopausal syndrome (1). Of these, about 35% go to their doctors requesting medical treatment. The following list shows the prevalence of symptoms in 380 women attending a menopause research clinic (2). It includes both those symptoms that are generally supposed to be due to low oestrogen levels, judged by the effectiveness of HRT in treating them, and those that do not seem to be so related.

Symptoms	*Per cent*
Hot flushes and sweats	84
Lethargy	73
Depression, anxiety, irritability	67
Reduced libido (sex urge)	65
Insomnia (broken sleep)	61
Headaches	61
Hair/skin changes	58
Poor memory/concentration	57
Painful intercourse	52
Dry vagina	46
Loss of confidence	46
Loss of femininity	31
Urinary symptoms	28
Oral (i.e. mouth) symptoms	26

There are a number of theories about the cause of menopausal symptoms, although no one is as yet quite certain why they occur. In order to understand what is known about them, it is easiest to consider them under the three headings of the main disturbances involved.

1 VASCULAR DISTURBANCE

Hot flushes, night sweats and occasional palpitations are thought to be due to a faulty mechanism within the hypothalamus area of the brain. The 'vasomotor centre' of the hypothalamus normally functions as a reflex centre controlling the calibre of peripheral blood vessels. In this way, the small 'peripheral' vessels in the skin are dilated or constricted according to our requirements. A warm environment causes them to dilate, giving the skin a pink appearance and enabling the blood to be cooled as it is brought nearer to the surface. A cold environment has the opposite effect.

When this reflex control is upset, blood vessels in the skin – particularly that of the face, neck and upper chest – dilate inappropriately, producing a hot flush. The colour of the face usually – although not always – becomes noticeably pinker as a result, and profuse sweating all over the body can occur as well, especially in bed at night.

It has been suggested that this lack of control is in some way connected with the increased output of FSH (follicle stimulating hormone) from the pituitary gland (see Chapter One). Another theory is that it coincides with a 'flushing band' of blood oestrogen levels peculiar in range to each woman, above and below which control is normal.

Regardless of its cause, the resultant hot flush can cause much embarrassment and discomfort. The night sweats, too, produce disturbed sleep both for the woman and frequently for her partner. In addition, the rate of the heart increases by about 20 beats/minute. Awareness of an increased heart beat without realizing the reason, can cause much needless worry about underlying heart disease.

Hot flushes and sweats generally last for a few minutes. They can occur rarely, or several times within an hour. Night sweats seem to come on without a stimulus, but day time hot flushes can be triggered by alcohol, hot or spicy food and drink, or an overheated room. The function of the hypothalamus is affected by the feelings and emotions, and hot flush attacks are closely related to stress and emotional upsets.

2 MEMBRANE CHANGES

This refers to the 'shrivelling' or degeneration of the membranous tissue lining the urethra (bladder outlet), and the vagina, in some menopausal women.

In the developing embryo, part of the bladder named the 'trigone', the upper part of the urethra, and the upper part of the vagina are all derived from a common structure named the Mullerian duct. This helps to explain why their lining membranes (or epithelium) react similarly to the diminishing blood level of oestrogen as ovarian function declines. The 'urethral syndrome' arises in some women as a result, with symptoms which are often misdiagnosed as cystitis. They include 'frequency' (i.e. increased frequency in passing urine, both during the day time and at night), pain on passing urine ('dysuria'), and sometimes 'haematuria' — blood in the urine. When the need to pass urine several times during the night is combined with night sweats, the resulting sleep disturbance can be severe.

Other possible urinary symptoms include urgency (the need to get to a lavatory without delay once the need to pass urine is felt); and urge incontinence, which refers to the involuntary passage of urine when urgency is experienced.

When the lining membrane of the vagina degenerates, the results are vaginal dryness; and an increased proneness to vaginal infections (for example, the yeast infection 'thrush', or bacterial infections). The corrugated, distensible vaginal lining membrane loses its folds and as a result, the vagina is less capable of stretching and expansion. This decrease in internal 'room' and the lack of adequate lubrication can combine to make intercourse a painful experience.

It should be said in this connection that loss of libido (sex drive) has usually been attributed in the past to uncomfortable intercourse. This may in fact be so. But some authorities claim that libido loss in itself is an important feature of the menopausal syndrome (2). Certainly the above table suggests that this symptom is much commoner (65%) than either 'dry vagina' (46%) or 'painful intercourse' (52%). And it is pointed out by the same author, that although some women with libido loss do respond to HRT, many will respond 'only to the addition of testosterone (male sex hormone) to the therapy'.

This finding supports the theory that there is a specific loss of sex drive, since the addition of testosterone would not be required to produce an improvement if membrane changes due to oestrogen lack were the only underlying cause.

Vaginal and urinary symptoms due to membrane changes tend to occur at a later stage of the menopause than the hot flushes and sweats due to vascular disturbance. They are sometimes accompanied by changes in the skin lining the vulva, the external genital area lying between the outer lips (labia majora).

Some women experience extreme itching (pruritus vulvae), which is both distressing and embarrassing. Others develop a condition known as kraurosis vulvae, in which the vulval area becomes dry, inflamed and painful. This condition requires prompt treatment, both for the relief of discomfort and because it predisposes to infections and possibly to malignant disease at a later date.

3 PSYCHOLOGICAL PROBLEMS

Both the vascular disturbances and the membrane changes discussed above, have been shown by properly conducted trials with menopausal patients (2) to respond well to oestrogen therapy. They are therefore attributed to menopausal oestrogen deficiency, but there is evidence to show that many other significant factors exist as well.

As I mentioned in Chapter One, the busier you are, the less likely you are to experience menopausal problems. Or, to quote Leon Chaitow, well-known osteopathic and naturopathic expert, writing on this topic in *Here's Health* magazine (4): 'It is well established that professional women, and those active outside the home, have fewer and less severe menopausal problems than housewives in general, especially those in low income groups. This indicates that factors other than purely hormonal ones are involved.'

Orthodox authorities find it less easy to relate emotional and psychological problems occurring during the 'change' to a lack of oestrogen. They are rarely improved by a course of oestrogen supplementation unless hot flushes, vaginal soreness and/or night sweats are also present.

Placebo-controlled clinical studies of women with severe oestrogen deficiency symptoms (5) have indicated that relief from vascular disturbances results in the relief of anxiety, irritability and worry about getting old. This is often combined with increased self-confidence, improved memory, and better powers of concentration. It is therefore believed that in the majority of cases, emotional and psychological problems arise as a result of, rather than independently of, the other menopausal symptoms. It is a mistake, however, to attribute all anxiety and depression arising in menopausal women to hot flushes and membrane soreness.

Both men and women with a tendency to neurotic illness, are more likely to develop signs and symptoms of it under conditions of stress. The middle years are known to impose a number of severe stresses on many of us, unless we take steps to protect ourselves in advance from their ill effects. There also seems to be an inherent tendency for depression to occur in middle and old age.

Recent epidemiological studies carried out at the Manchester Royal Infirmary, for example, and reported on by Doctor Madeline Osborn in 1984, failed to show a clear link between depression and the menopause (6). Professor Martin Vessey and his colleagues in Oxford, on the other hand, found from answers to a postal questionnaire sent to 809 women on GP lists that psychiatric symptoms were associated more with chronological age than with the menopause (7).

Doctor Osborn referred in her research paper to another Oxford study (unpublished at the time of her writing), in which 521 women between the ages of 35 and 59 were interviewed. Women whose periods had stopped in the previous year, were no more likely to be psychiatrically ill than women who were still menstruating.

On the other hand, women in the 45 to 49 year age group who suffered from vascular disturbances, were far more likely to develop psychiatric symptoms than women without symptoms.

Despite this association, attempts to treat depressed menopausal women with oestrogens generally produced discouraging results.

BONE THINNING (OSTEOPOROSIS)

A certain amount of bone thinning affects everyone, and begins around the age of twenty years. Osteoporosis (an advanced stage of bone thinning) develops when the process is accelerated, and this occurs in a variety of conditions, including overactivity of the thyroid gland, rheumatoid arthritis, Cushing's syndrome (over-activity of the adrenal glands) and – in some women – the menopause.

Menopausal osteoporosis appears to be directly related to oestrogen deficiency, since supplemental oestrogen treats the condition successfully and is often suggested as a preventive measure against its development. There is, however, much con-troversy, even among the orthodox medical profession, about the part played by other factors, in particular inadequate diet, insuf-ficient exercise, and stress factors.

A well-known expert in this field, Dr A. Fowler, of Bridgend General Hospital (8) in Wales, had the following comment to make in a letter to the *British Medical Journal*: 'If the post-menopausal woman is an active exerciser, does not smoke, and eats oily fish or has moderate exposure to sunlight, she is unlikely to suffer from appreciable osteoporosis.'

The effect of osteoporosis on bone is essentially loss of density. The bones remain roughly the same size in outline, but there is a gradual loss of the organic structure (matrix) from which they are formed, accompanied by a loss of calcium salts with which the matrix is impregnated. In very severe cases, the yearly loss (1) can amount to 2% of cortical bone (the outer hard shell), and 7% of 'spongy' bone (the bone's interior structure). Put another way, by the time she reaches her seventieth birthday, a woman can have lost 50% of her total bone mass, in contrast to a man who, by the age of 95, will on average have lost only 25%.

The effects of osteoporosis are not apparent at the time of the menopause. The diagnosis is usually made on X-rays performed for some other reason, and it is not until middle age has been left well behind that osteoporosis can be detected on the grounds of symptoms. One of these is increased bone brittleness. This greatly increases the risk of fractures – the most significant of which is fractured neck of femur (the upper end of the long thigh bone).

The cost of this fracture to the NHS every year is more than £100 million, and to the patient, a greatly increased chance of death. It is the typical injury sustained by elderly women as a result of tripping over an uneven kerb, or slipping down on icy pavements in the winter. Fifteen per cent of all elderly patients sustaining this injury die within three months.

Not all women develop a serious degree of osteoporosis after their menopause, and there is no way of telling whether you are likely or unlikely to be affected. Certain groups (1) of post-menopausal women are known to have an increased risk. These include women who have undergone a premature menopause (i.e. before the age of 40); thin women (because, having less fat, they synthesize less oestrogen from precursor substances – p. 3 above); and women with several family members who are sufferers.

Besides fractured neck of femur, osteoporosis can cause aches and pains in the back and limbs; shortening of the spine, leading to loss of height and a rounded upper back; and vertebral collapse, causing sudden severe pain in the affected back area.

HORMONE REPLACEMENT THERAPY

We saw in the last chapter that the single most important bio-chemical change occurring at the menopause is the falling level of ovarian 'oestradiol'. We have also seen in this chapter, that while certain menopausal symptoms seem to be closely related to this factor (e.g. night sweats, hot flushes, membrane degeneration), others seem to be less so. These latter include depression, irritability, headaches, poor memory and concentration, joint and muscular aches and pains, and are apt to arise rather as a reaction to the hormone-related symptoms than as a direct result of hormonal change.

At least with respect to the oestrogen-deficient problems, ortho-dox doctors feel that the best possible solution is oestrogen supplementation (HRT). The problem that arose at first in con-nection with this approach, was that women treated in this way had an increased risk of developing womb cancer (uterine car-cinoma).

Although this risk has now been minimized (see below), hor-mone replacement therapy has never entirely lost its image as a dangerous form of treatment. This perturbs many doctors who feel that the possible risks of HRT have been wildly exaggerated, and that many women suffer unnecessarily because they are afraid to accept treatment that can in fact be practically guaranteed to work.

Partly because it is currently fashionable to prefer alternative forms of therapy, and partly because of the real if slight risk involved, orthodox doctors have been severely criticized for their support of HRT. They are castigated as being culpably ignorant, and indifferent to their patients' welfare. Their critics seem to believe that prescriptions for HRT are dashed off with a blithe lack of concern about the risks involved, and largely for the ultimate profit of the pharmaceutical companies with whom doctors are surely in league!

That this is not at all the case can be seen in the controversy that continues to permeate every aspect of the topic whenever it is raised. Read what the following consultant gynaecologist, Doctor Louis Goldman, has to say about bone thinning and oestrogen prevention therapy (9):

'Can we prevent osteoporosis and, if we can, what are the risks? Merely to ask the question is to bring us face to face with what I once described as the Four Horsemen of the Medical Apoc-alypse – confusion, contradiction, uncertainty and paradox.

'No one questions that the long-term administration of oestrogen protects women from the bone loss associated with the post-menopausal state, and there is at least presumptive evidence (from case-control studies) that it also reduces the risk of fracture. Trying to balance these advantages against the risks, however, immediately creates problems. And dogmatic assurances, even from experts who have studied osteoporosis for years, do not take us very far.'

Of course HRT has its committed supporters. Dr J. M. Aitken of Essex County Hospital expressed the following views in the *British Medical Journal*, in November 1984 (3): doctors 'should stop frightening women with the imaginary evils of hormone replacement treatment.'

He pointed out that cancer fears have resulted in fewer than 2% of patients being willing to accept HRT. He felt that the preconditions (frequent pelvic examinations and womb scrapes) imposed on prospective recipients were sufficiently off-putting to deter the majority of them. He labelled as false the 'grim forebodings of the prophets of doom', and stated that there is no good evidence that intermittent oestrogen treatment is associated with any real risk of genital cancer. He felt that womb scrapes were only necessary in women who experienced unexplained bleeding.

He recommended the combined use of both oestradiol and synthetic progesterone – the first to be used for twenty-one days of the cycle, and the second to be used on the seven oestrogen-free days. This he suggested was a natural way of treating ovarian hormone deficiency, and the most effective way of reducing the prevalence of osteoporosis. He commented that, instead of frightening women about HRT, 'we should start to woo them with the possible long term benefits.'

The most obvious question that arises is, how has such confusion arisen in the first place? Either HRT involves a risk of cancer, or it does not, so how can different opinions exist over a point that is either true or false? Unfortunately, the problem is not clear-cut, and it is impossible to reply in terms of absolute certainty in view of the many differing reports that have been received from researchers in this field.

When oestrogens were first used for treating the menopause they were prescribed 'cyclically', i.e. on a regular basis or cycle of three out of every four weeks. Given in this way, they were found to overstimulate the womb lining (endometrium) into a condition called hyperplasia, meaning the excessive growth of normal cells. The hyperplastic cells bled every month during the oestrogen-free days, producing what is called a 'withdrawal bleed' due to the temporary absence of the hormone.

Hyperplasia of the womb lining is a benign (non-cancerous) condition, but one which merits careful watching. Cancer is also 'excessive growth' -- but with one vital difference. Cancerous cells subdivide and multiply wildly, in a completely ungoverned fashion. Hyperplastic cells retain their basic self-control, but 'go overboard' in developing with far more vigour than is usual for them. Very occasionally, hyperplastic tissue cells lose self-control, and become cancerous.

Hyperplasia of the womb lining occurred in about 30% of the women treated in the early days with cyclical oestrogens, within two years of the start of treatment (10). In a small percentage of women receiving this treatment, endometrial cancer subsequently developed (11). The cancer risk now appears to have been minimized by adding a progestogen to the oestrogen therapy for at least twelve days per calendar month (10,12).

Despite this, women taking a course of oestrogen/progestogen still have a withdrawal bleed (1) during or just after the days of the month on which progestogen is taken. This indicates that the endometrium is still stimulated into a hyperplastic condition, although the progestogen part of the treatment is known to offer 'maximum protection' against malignancy.

The actual size of the present degree of risk is difficult to assess with certainty. It depends entirely upon which research papers you read. Many different figures are obtained, some suggesting the risk to be definitely present but 'low', while others find that the risk is infinitesimally small.

An argument sometimes put forward on behalf of HRT, is that the combined therapy now used actually protects women against certain forms of cancer. The cancer concerned, though, is not *womb* cancer, but *breast* cancer. This is a point that many of

HRT's supporters fail to make clear. A risk still exists – albeit a small one – of cancer of the womb resulting from HRT. The progestogens now included in the treatment simply afford 'maximum protection' against this risk (i.e. they minimize it to the greatest degree possible at present).

Complications

Before we leave the subject of HRT, it is only fair to mention the contraindications to taking it. HRT is absolutely contraindicated (except under very rare circumstances) in the presence of any form of cancer likely to be affected by oestrogen (e.g. cancer of breast, cervix, uterus). Relative contraindications to its use include previous hyperplasia of the womb lining, thrombosis (clot formation) involving arteries or veins, a pre-existing raised blood pressure, and diabetes (1).

Studies of the fat and cholesterol levels in the blood are advised before prescribing HRT for any woman with a family history of arterial disease (for example, coronary heart disease), although not all blood lipid (i.e. fat) abnormalities are contraindications to HRT. An example of one that does contraindicate its use is hypertriglyceridaemia, which is an abnormally raised blood level of fats of the triglyceride family.

Women who have had problems with blood clot formation, need careful blood clotting studies performed before receiving oestrogen. Specialist consultation is also advisable, generally speaking, in diabetic patients whose stable condition might be adversely affected by HRT. In addition, patients with high blood pressure need to have this problem sorted out and brought under control before commencing treatment.

Finally, few doctors would prescribe HRT for women who suffered from severe varicose veins, benign breast disease or active or oestrogen-related liver disease. Women who smoke heavily, who are very overweight, or who have gallstones also stand a greater risk than others of complications developing.

HRT versus natural methods

That HRT has many supporters, including satisfied patients, is unarguable. No one would deny the advantages of avoiding osteoporosis and the increased risk of fractures in old age, or undervalue relief from vaginal and urethral membrane degeneration. Nevertheless, a high percentage of menopausal women refuse treatment on the grounds of increased cancer risk, and put up with the health problems involved rather than having to worry whether *they* might be one of the few unlucky ones. They are the women who are well aware that the 'slight risk' involved means, in fact, 'slightly increased risk'. All women with a uterus run some risk of getting endometrial cancer, simply because this is a change that the lining of the uterus is prone under certain conditions to undergo. Taking supplementary sex hormones increases this risk – in however slight a way – at the very age at which this form of cancer is most likely, statistically, to develop. There seems very little justification for this, in view of the fact that other, drug-free methods can achieve the same end without any risks whatever.

The remaining chapters of this book describe this natural approach to the menopause, both curative and preventive. The oestrogen-deficiency symptoms respond very well to a number of drug-free forms of treatment, and the non-oestrogen related ones can also be avoided or relieved. In every instance, the measures I recommend are absolutely safe, and you need have no fear that they might be contraindicated in your case, or that complications or side effects might result.

Chapter Three

Food for pleasure – and energy

So much real scientific and technological progress has been made since the beginning of the century, that it can come as a shock to realize how much of value has been lost. Far from being confined to a retrogressive over-forties minority, this opinion is shared – and perpetrated – in several important respects by leading experts in many fields. The particular respect of interest to us here, is that of nutrition.

So much is written on the subject, in fact, that the very word is likely to provoke the image of an overloaded bandwagon, on which dozens of enthusiastic diet reformers are competing for standing room. In fact, an old-fashioned scene of a pitched battle would be more appropriate. One army flies the (dun-coloured?) flag of wholefood dietary reform, while the other unashamedly flaunts the brilliantly artificial colours of the processed food industry.

Among the champions of the first, we note nutritional experts such as Professor John Yudkin, Dr Hugh Sinclair, Dr Alec Forbes and Adele Davis, and rank upon rank of writers, broadcasters, health magazine editors, alternative medicine professionals and diet reform converts. Leaders of the opposing field include heads of the sugar, flour, processed foods, confectionery and food additive industries, and executives of the Milk Marketing Board, the Butter Council, and the Ministry for Agriculture and Fisheries.

Bringing up the rear guard are all the purveyors of fast snacks, sweets and processed foods, and all the advertising executives engaged in making poor quality food as irresistible as possible.

There is little need to comment on the victories gained by the industrial giants. Hundreds of gallons of chemically coloured fruit squash and fizzy drinks, tons of tasteless, sliced white loaves, and mountains of greasy chips deluged in lurid sauces are consumed with relish every day of the year in this country. Together, of course, with sky-high piles of frozen hamburgers and sausages, hundreds of packets of refined white sugar and many hundred-weights of chocolate, synthetically flavoured sweets and icecream.

However, to win a battle, or even a sequence of battles, is nothing like winning a war, and there are signs that the urgent warnings of the nutritional experts are getting through to us. During 1984, skimmed milk sales more than trebled, and whole milk consumption fell from an average 3.84 pints per person per week, to 3.61 pints (13). Sales of pork, beef, veal, lamb, eggs and sugar were also reduced. The national consumption of poultry rose, however, and the national average consumption stands at 7.7 ounces per week. Other sales increases included brown and wholemeal bread, fruit juices and breakfast cereals. Sales of fresh fruit and vegetables were down, though.

You may well be wondering what all this has to do with the menopause, and why the above trends in national eating habits should be such good news. Research has shown that certain types of food are clearly linked with a number of diseases common in our society, and nutritional experts are doing their best to spread the news of recent findings.

Discussion of a representative selection would require a chapter in itself, but I will mention a few of the more familiar disease-and-dietary links which have been established. Best known is, perhaps, heart and arterial disease, which are linked with a high intake of saturated animal fat. Obesity is clearly linked with too great an intake of energy in the form of food calories.

Refined sugar provides 'empty' calories without supplying any necessary nourishment, and dietary fat supplies more than twice the calorific energy that either protein or carbohydrate supplies, weight for weight.

Diverticulitis (small, inflamed herniations of colon lining membrane that project through the large bowel wall) is connected with too little dietary fibre. Colonic cancer is also linked with a low roughage diet – and probably with chemical additives used to flavour and preserve meat, and with a high intake of red meat, especially beef and its fat.

Diabetes is believed to be precipitated by the habit of swamping the bloodstream with sugar, by eating large quantities of refined sugar snacks, especially in childhood. In addition, poor return of vein blood from the lower limbs (and the resultant varicose veins) are associated with too much sugar and fat, and especially with too little fibre.

Finally, high blood pressure is aggravated in some people by a high sodium intake – we eat a great deal more salt than the body requires. Benign (i.e. non-cancerous) breast disease is linked with coffee-drinking, hyperactivity in some children with the chemical additives in processed foods, heavy tea-drinking with peptic ulcers and – recently discovered – lung cancer with (besides tobacco smoke) a high intake of dietary cholesterol.

Inevitably, information of this type is spread in the face of mighty opposition from powerful food industry moguls. They do their best to spread the idea of nutritional experts (especially those qualified in alternative therapies) as unreliable, freakish scaremongers with their own vested interests to care for.

There is another reason why the recent trends towards healthier eating in this country are such good news. The new nutritional wisdom is far from purely negative. The right diet makes for positive health and well-being, and there is all the difference in the world between not suffering from any specific disorder, and feeling physically and mentally on top of the world. The better your general state of health, the less likely you are to fall prey to major or minor ills, current infections, chronic fatigue, depression and anxiety.

Added bonuses of healthy eating include improved performance in sports, more 'staying power' for busy mothers, housewives and working women, loss of surplus weight without deliberately 'going on a diet', and – even more important if you are overweight now — the maintenance of your newly gained slim figure. Further benefits in this direction are the effects of good food on your looks. Many people find that their hair grows more thickly and gains body and lustre, and that their complexions become clear and early wrinkles less noticeable. Skin, in particular, seems to benefit. Instead of hanging in sagging folds due to weight loss, its elasticity is retained and it 'fits' without telltale signs of previous excess weight.

Besides benefiting from positive good health and looks, many women discover that menstrual problems improve beyond measure and sometimes even disappear altogether. A diet with a high percentage of raw food (which I will discuss a little later) is particularly renowned for helping irregular, heavy or painful periods, and menopausal symptoms — especially hot flushes — have also been greatly relieved.

Healthy Eating and the Menopause

Consider then, the possible benefits you could gain from eating healthily, if you are suffering from menopausal symptoms or are out to prevent such symptoms from arising in the first place. Many experts (and I subscribe to this view) deny that any physiological reason exists for women to put on weight and develop a middle-age spread, either at, or after, the menopause. Exercise and diet are major causative factors, and these can be eliminated once you know how to set about it. The diet I will describe will be an enormous asset in this direction.

In addition, increased staying power and improved ability to cope with stress could surely never be of more value to you than at the present time. Add to this improved memory and concentration, freedom from minor headaches, aches and pains, and an increased sense of calm and tranquillity, together with a more youthful appearance, and you will not need convincing that if a diet can achieve all this, it should be followed carefully.

WHOLEFOOD EATING

What precisely *is* this diet that bestows such a multitude of benefits? It is simply a 'wholefood' diet, consisting of foods from which nothing has been taken away, and to which nothing has been added. It is food of very much the same quality as that which our great-grandparents ate, tempered only by our greater knowledge of the biochemical significance of animal and plant protein, carbohydrate, fats, minerals and vitamins.

Besides the lack of additions and subtractions, wholefoods are not processed or refined in any way. This means that they are not subjected to abnormally high temperatures, or to chemical treatments such as sulphur dioxide preservation (some dried fruit) or hydrogenation (some margarines) in its preparation. Wholefoods are also free from all artificial colouring matter, preservatives, flavourings, thickeners and emulsifiers. Because of this, they are less likely to trigger abnormal behaviour in children, and mysterious symptoms such as frequent headaches, digestive upsets, diarrhoea and constipation, which are sometimes caused by unsuspected food allergies. Some experts even feel that chemical food additives may help to generate cancer.

Some people object that wholefoods must be boring, and slow and fiddly to prepare. After all, (they think), wholefood eating automatically precludes popping into the nearest Wimpy or McDonald's while out shopping, and probably even pubs and restaurants as well. Certainly the first two pose problems, but when you have spent some time eating natural foods only, packet soups, white baps (even with sesame seeds on top) containing beefburgers of unfathomable origin, and bright red and green knickerbocker glories lose their old appeal.

Pubs and restaurants are a different matter. Pubs by and large are able to offer a selection of salads with hard boiled eggs, cheese, chicken or cold fish (avoid the battered cod fried in a vat of reheated oil), and are often able to produce brown or wholemeal bread as an accompaniment. And wholefood enthusiasts are certainly not against a moderate intake of alcohol! A glass of dry white wine is pleasantly refreshing on a hot day, and certain real ales contain nutriments of value to health.

Restaurants are an even better bet. Choose melon, grapefruit or freshly squeezed fruit juice, grilled white fish or chicken, lightly boiled or steamed vegetables, a brown unbuttered roll and fresh fruit or water ice as a dessert, and you have eaten a meal that should be easy to select from the vast majority of menus in this country. Even more important, your choice will be indistinguishable from that of your non-wholefooder companions, who are likely to choose cholesterol and sugar-rich foods, and add unconsciously to their daily intake of colouring matter, preservatives, chemical flavourings and other additives.

Whether or not you decide to try converting *them* to wholefood depends very much on your relationship with them! But if you are patient with your own new way of eating for a couple of months, you are very likely to find that other people ask you to share your new health and beauty secrets.

When I said that wholefood eating has much in common with the dietary patterns of our great-grandparents, I did not have in mind endless dishes of boiled mutton and steak and kidney pie, baked rice puddings and semolina with prunes. These are very nice in their way and it is possible to cook them according to healthy recipes. But the emphasis was upon 'wholesome, plain' food — a phrase which is very much misunderstood these days. Wholefood is plain in the sense that it is uncontaminated by chemicals; and wholesome in the sense that much of it is either eaten raw or lightly cooked and fresh from the garden or shops. By running through a typical day's menus I will give you an idea of the variety and appeal of many of the dishes. The meals described here also comply closely with the wholefood diet of benefit to menopausal women, which Leon Chaitow (consultant naturopath and osteopath) described in his article on this subject in the November 1983 issue of *Here's Health* magazine.

Breakfast
Most people find cereals and bread or toast acceptable and

convenient to prepare in the morning. Try wholewheat flakes or wholegrain cereal, which retain their germ of life and their natural fibre. There is no need to sprinkle added bran on this sort of breakfast food. Eat it with a little fresh fruit and fruit juice, or add skimmed milk.

If you have a sweet tooth, choose a muesli which provides sweetness by containing a reasonable proportion of natural, dried fruits such as dates, figs, raisins and slices of apple or banana, rather than added sugar. Delicious additions are fresh, live yoghurt, and a sprinkling of sunflower or pumpkin seeds. For menopausal symptoms, the live yoghurt helps to protect a dry vagina from thrush infection. The sunflower seeds have a natural sedative that brings calm and tranquillity when you feel irritated and het up, but is completely non-addictive.

Skimmed milk is preferable to full cream milk (one of the rare food items with 'something taken away' that wholefooders do include in their diets!) because of the low saturated fat content. This helps protect your heart and arteries, and reduces your calorie intake at the same time.

If you find you miss fried bacon and eggs, try a lightly boiled free-range egg instead. Accompany this with a slice or two of wholemeal (preferably whole grain) bread or toast, and avoid plastic-wrapped, ready sliced white bread. Either eat your slice of wholegrain bread dry (make sure it's very fresh), or spread with a little margarine that is high in polyunsaturated fats. A popular choice is Vitaquell, despite the unfortunate brand name chosen for it!

Don't drink tea or coffee. Both contain stimulants to which you can become addicted, and while tea is associated with peptic ulcer formation, coffee is possibly associated with an increased risk of stomach cancer, and has definitely been linked with benign disease of the breast. Substitute fresh fruit juice (more about that later) or, if you need something hot, try a herbal or fruit tea.

It was with great reluctance that I allowed myself to be persuaded to try one of these teas recently, because I detest ordinary tea and couldn't believe that these would not resemble it in some way. I was delighted to discover that this was not the case, and now drink either apple tea or the 'bright and early' Secret Garden blend made by the London Herb and Spice Company, which contains orange peel, cherry rind, rosehip, blackberry leaves, spearmint, lemon grass and hibiscus flowers.

Lunch (interchangeable with dinner)
Aim to eat a salad at lunch time, either as a packed meal which you take to work, or at home where you can keep the ingredients cool in the fridge until you feel like preparing them. This ensures that you are taking a fair percentage of your daily food in its raw state (see 'Raw foods' below), and the variety available is enormous.

Use leafy vegetables, including grated raw cabbage, raw spinach or broccoli, grated sprouts (which are excellent) and chopped or grated celery and root vegetables such as beetroot, carrots, young turnips, swedes or parsnips. Use tomatoes, spring onions, cucumber, lettuce and radishes when they are available in good condition, and don't feel a salad is not one without them.

Add to your daily salad base a few seeds, some chopped nuts (not too many if you are dieting), some sprouted seeds (alfalfa, mung bean, fenugreek are all easily available through health food shops). Eat with this some fresh cottage or low fat curd cheese, a boiled egg if you haven't already had one for breakfast, a little grated Edam or Gouda, and a baked jacket potato of which you should eat the skin.

You can add a slice of wholemeal bread or toast; or, as a change, you can experiment with grains you may not have tried before. Wholegrain rice is probably familiar, and is certainly delicious, either hot or cold, especially when cooked until only just firm (about twenty minutes). Add a low sodium salt substitute if you like, and a few herbs, or a little grated onion, slivers of garlic or a small knob of margarine.

Less familiar grains are wheat, barley, burgur wheat, millet and buckwheat. These are all very pleasant, and help to provide you with plenty of choice. I especially enjoy whole barley grains simmered with a little Vecon, a strong, delicious vegetable extract not unlike Marmite, and used for flavouring stocks, soups and casseroles.

Dinner

Include your main protein item at this meal, and choose from white fish, oily fish such as mackerel, herring, fresh sardines or pilchards, kidney or liver, poultry or game, or a vegetarian savoury. The oily fish supplies certain vital fatty acids which help maintain a healthy heart and arteries. They also supply vitamin D, which you need for the maintenance of healthy bone structure. Among the oily fish, grilled herring with mustard are delicious and so are fresh mackerel or fresh sardines. Among the white fish, try lightly cooked plaice, cod or coley, casseroled or steamed, and flavoured with tomato, a little onion or garlic, or some fresh or dried herbs. Dried dill weed is very tasty, and so is sweet basil.

Accompany your protein with lots of lightly cooked (steamed or stir-fried) vegetables, a baked potato if you want one, and follow with a dessert of fresh fruit, plain live yoghourt, or a fresh fruit salad, fruit water ice or crumble (if you are not dieting). Make the crumble top with wholemeal flour and margarine, and a *little* demerara, barbados or muscovado sugar and some cinnamon, nutmeg or powdered ginger if you like them. Use wholewheat flour and margarine when you make pastry; and try making your own bread with wholegrain flour and live yeast. Its flavour is so superior to that of the factory-baked product that you are likely to make a habit of making your own.

Leon Chaitow (4) suggests that alcohol intake should be limited by women suffering from (or trying to avoid) menopausal symptoms to two glasses of wine or their equivalent daily. This is a good idea, particularly if you suffer from hot flushes which are often made worse by tippling. If you are used to more than this amount daily, or find that you crave for extra drink when you feel irritable and low, explore the unfamiliar and try freshly squeezed fruit or vegetable juices. An electric juice extractor is the gadget you need, and having acquired one you will probably find yourself using it every day. Fruit juices are delightful alone, or can be used to dilute either your daily wine allowance or equivalent in spirits (two single measures).

Carrot juice has an unjustified aura of crankiness about it, although I cannot think how it arose, unless it was from its connection with Doctor Barbara More in the 'fifties, who walked, so I understand, right across the United States relying almost entirely upon the nourishment provided by this particular juice. She seems to have done very well on the strength of it and, apart from its vitality-promoting properties, it is quite delicious, being sweet and rich-tasting, and creamy in consistency. Nevertheless, I know the proprietors of one famous health farm who refuse to serve it in case they get labelled as health cranks!

Other unexpectedly delicious juices include beetroot, also rich and sweet; radish — but take in small quantities only as it is very strong; and apple. Carrot juice is very rich in vitamin A, and also supplies vitamins B, C, D, E and K. Beetroot juice supplies vitamins A, B1 and C, and iron (useful if your periods have been heavy). Radish juice provides vitamins B1 and C, and is rich in potassium, sodium, iron and magnesium. Combined with carrot juice, it 'soothes and heals mucous membranes' (14). Apple juice provides vitamins A, B1 and C, and potassium, sodium and phosphorus (a constituent of bone), it is very good for the complexion, and aids the breakdown of dietary fat.

The following juices are recommended by raw juice therapy expert Bridget Amies to promote health and strength: equal parts of carrot and grape juice, and one teaspoonful of radish juice. Take 4 ounces slowly before meals.

John B. Lust, one of the best known names in the recent history of raw juice therapy, suggests that carrot juice taken in the afternoon (try half a pint) 'helps to keep the mucous membranes, glands, bones, walls of the arteries, in fact the entire body in healthy condition' (14). Also that celery juice taken before retiring is 'soothing, relaxing, alleviates anxiety and worry and promotes restful sleep.' Celery juice is a natural nerve tonic and is high in calcium (very important for healthy bones), phosphorus, sodium and potassium. It aids the body to utilize calcium supplies as it should, and it helps arthritic conditions.

Both carrot and celery juice, therefore, have considerable application to menopausal symptoms.

I referred at the beginning of the chapter to 'health food converts' – mainly because changing from an 'ordinary' diet to a wholefood one requires forethought and determination, and people have to be pretty convinced of the benefits of such a change to make the effort required. It is essential, though, to remember that wholefood eating is a better and healthier way of life, and not a religion with a plethora of dogmas demanding total compliance at all times.

There are bound to be occasions – for instance, at dinner parties, meals provided by relatives, or outings from work or with a club – where the menu is set and you have no opportunity to choose what you eat. My advice is simply do the best you can, and eat the food provided rather than offend your host and hostess. You can always ask for small portions of, say, boeuf en croute or commercially prepared shepherd's pie, accept a minimum of chips, and help yourself to as large a portion of frozen sprouts, peas or spinach as would be considered polite!

I do not, on the whole, advocate trying to persuade other people to join you in your new eating habits. When they are your guests, the chances are that they will not even notice any difference in the kind of meals you prepare – until it comes to the dessert, perhaps.

They might raise an eyebrow at your fresh blackberry water ice or yoghourt-based apricot syllabub replacing old favourites such as 'naughty but nice' fresh cream cakes, or spotted dick and custard. But if you do explain about wholefood eating, be prepared for a certain amount of jokes made at your expense, and the expense of the health food industry and alternative medical practitioners generally.

Many people are afraid of change and feel threatened by it – and you will probably find that they categorically deny that there is any sensible foundation for, say, reducing their intake of sugar or animal fat. This attitude is maintained by some people, despite the massive amount of evidence that exists for these items endangering our health, much as addicted smokers (say they) refuse to believe in the link between arterial and heart disease, lung cancer and tobacco smoke.

With respect to your nearest and dearest, do remember to make the change gradually. If you happen to live alone, and *feel* like discarding processed and over-refined foods overnight, that is entirely your affair. But to serve up locally bought battered cod and chips, followed by tinned fruit salad and icecream one week, and expect cries of enthusiasm to greet grilled plaice, jacket potatoes and a large side salad decorated with pumpkin seeds the next, is asking too much of the most uncritical family.

'Softee, softee, catchee monkey' is the motto – do it gradually and DON'T DISCUSS IT! If you introduce changes subtly enough, for instance changing from sliced white bread to sliced wrapped wholemeal and gradually making your own, using only 81% wholemeal flour in the early stages, the chances are high that no one will notice. If you are asked about the changes you are making – whatever you do, don't say it's to help relieve you of menopausal symptoms! The benefits I have outlined in this respect are yours for the taking, and so is far more enjoyable and satisfying food into the bargain. But people (even families) start to feel deprived if you talk about nutritious meals before they have discovered how good they are, and unnecessary arguments can arise.

(81% wholemeal flour, by the way, is the whole grain milled into flour which includes all the wheatgerm, but which has a proportion of the bran extracted to make it lighter in colour and less of a change from the artificially bleached 'white'.)

RAW FOODS

Once you are used to planning and preparing wholefood menus, there are two improvements you can make. The first is to 'buy organic' as much as possible – or even better, grow your own without artificial crop fertilizers and pest controllers – since the value of any fruit or vegetables depends ultimately upon the quality of the soil in which they were grown.

The farming industry opts for adding excessive amounts of nitrogenous compounds to the soil, and for spraying crops with chemicals to kill pests. This leaves a residue of possibly harmful (perhaps even cancer-producing) chemicals on and in the food we buy, and there is no way of knowing – yet – exactly what may be the long-term effects on us of this daily consumption of laboratory compounds.

The same goes for meat, poultry and eggs. Sheep and cattle, poultry and laying hens are given hormones, artificial food supplements and often antibiotics, in an attempt to hurry them and their products to the dinner table with the least possible trouble to the farmer and in the shortest possible time. The quality of their brief lives, and the manner in which they are put to death, is not something I have room to deal with here. But you will be doing yourself and your family a very good turn (and doubtless helping in the long run to influence society against inhumane animal treatment), by seeking out suppliers of organic, free-range meat, and free-range eggs.

The second refinement you can aim at is the inclusion of plenty of raw food in your daily diet. The remarkable best seller *Raw Energy* by Leslie and Susannah Kenton (23) offers a brilliant summary of much of the in-depth research carried out into the benefits of raw food eating.

Apart from offering tangible protection against various forms of cancer, relieving sufferers of chronic health problems, and actively assisting in the promotion of youthful beauty, raw foods provide specific help for a number of female health problems.

Leslie and Susannah suggest that eating about 75% raw foods daily is adequate for the desirable benefits to result. So much raw food, chiefly in the form of salads, would not suit everyone, either aesthetically or biochemically, but you might well find this way of eating – as I do – very appealing.

Here are some of the benefits special to women. As the authors point out, uncooked foods 'are one of the reasons why the world's exclusive and expensive health farms stay in business'.

- Iron, calcium, zinc and a variety of vitamin deficiencies are very common in women in our society. All the essential vitamins and minerals are vital for you to feel and look your best. Raw foods offer these, in the correctly balanced proportions, especially freshly squeezed vegetable juices and sprouted grains and seeds.
- Raw foods supply far more natural vitamin C and bioflavonoids (which are similar to a vitamin), and these keep collagen healthy. Collagen plays essential roles in skin, hair and nail health. Zinc stops stretch marks from forming when you lose weight. Vitamin A is present in abundance in raw foods and keeps the skin moist and of youthful texture.
- Cellulite disappears on a high-raw diet. This is encouraged by aerobic exercise and skin brushing, and by improved lymphatic drainage and stronger capillary structure (both of these due in part to the bioflavonoids in raw food).
- Monthly problems such as PMS (the premenstrual syndrome), bloating and fatigue tend to disappear after two or three months of high-raw eating. Periods get lighter. Again thanks are largely due to the bioflavonoids, as well as to carotene (a precursor of vitamin A), and to vitamin C.
- Menopausal hot flushes have been found to disappear.

These, then, are the advantages of wholefood eating and the inclusion of ample supplies of raw fruit and vegetables, nuts, grains and seeds in your diet.

We will now take a look at what else you can do to feel one hundred per cent on form from your forties onwards.

Chapter Four

Enjoying regular exercise

Hopefully, both the benefits of wholefood and high-raw eating – plus of course the foods themselves – will have convinced you that the flag flown by the supporters of natural eating, is anything but 'dun-coloured'. If you have thought in the past of wholemeal bread, brown rice and lentils as representative of wholefoods, you might well have made the error of regarding them as dreary rather than delicious. However, the brilliant array of reds, greens and oranges, tempered by beige, white and yellow that go to make up quite an ordinary salad of fresh fruit and vegetables in the huge variety of possible combinations, should convince you that dreariness is the last word that can be applied to wholefood, high-raw eating.

Regular exercise is another vital factor in your lifestyle, if you wish to become physically fit and make your menopause the start of a new lease of life. Like wholefoods, exercise is also badly misunderstood and misrepresented, and has an unattractive image among non-exercisers. Most people (men and women) who have not deliberately exercised for years, associate the word with painful, sweaty sessions in a gym (as seen on TV), and with joggers dropping like flies from heart attacks (as read about in newspaper and magazine articles).

One of the reasons for this misconception about exercise, is that people who are keen on jogging, swimming or cycling, naturally tend to share their interest with other enthusiasts, rather than preach the benefits of exercise to the determinedly unconverted. The staff of most offices or shop departments, for example, will have a cyclist, jogger or swimmer among them who pursues his or her daily exercise despite a lot of well-meaning jokes made by sedentary colleagues. All the latter see, in fact, is Sue or Joe arriving at work on a pouring wet day in cycling gear, or disappearing during the lunch hour with a rolled up towel under their arm. They just cannot know how enjoyable regular exercise can be (sporadic exercise is often a pain), nor how much better they would feel if they tried it for themselves.

So, what exactly are the benefits of keeping active when you are over forty – and how on earth do you start, when you haven't taken any proper exercise for twenty years or more?

To begin with, we saw from Dr Fowler's statement in Chapter Two, that 'active exercise' is one of the prerequisites in avoiding 'appreciable osteoporosis' (8). More specifically, it has been found to have a direct effect upon bone and calcium metabolism. Mark Bricklin, author of the *Practical Encyclopedia of Natural Healing*, sums up the important points in his chapter on exercise therapy.

'When we escape from hypokinesis (that is, inadequate physical activity), into the world of regular vigorous exercises, we are causing surprisingly profound changes in our physiology. The act of walking, for instance, combining both the exercise and the actual striking of the feet on a hard surface, *promotes the addition of minerals to bones*. That is apparently why astronauts, whose feet do not bump on any surfaces because of the absence of gravity, lose bone minerals despite dietary supplementation and exercise. *Regular long walks should be a part of the program of anyone hoping to prevent or arrest the progress of osteoporosis.*' (My italics.) (15)

Apart from the important factor of osteoporosis, exercise will help you with menopausal problems in the following ways:

- It combats the tendency to put on weight.
- It combats muscular aches and pains and stiffness, and discourages the development of arthritis.

- Rather than depleting you of what little energy you have, regular exercise increases your stamina and zest for living.
- It increases your expectation of life, by helping in a major way to protect you from heart and arterial disease, high blood pressure, and lung disease.
- It improves the quality of your life, by combating stress and nervous tension, and especially by fighting depression (post-menopausal blues).
- It improves your sex life! Regular exercise has the effect of an aphrodisiac on many men and women.

It is interesting to discover quite how exercise is capable of all these marvels.

1 We tend to put on weight when we are forty, because we live more sedentary lives than we did when we were twenty years younger. And instead of cutting down our food intake accordingly, we eat much the same as before.

There is no reason for us to become inactive so early in life – and as evidence of this, most of us know a hale and hearty septuagenarian or even octogenarian who still enjoys a competitive round of golf or a daily swim.

Instead of being inspired to exercise similarly, though, we talk about such individuals as though they were something quite out of the ordinary, and comment how marvellous they are 'for their age'. Actually, they're not, they are simply as fit as most of us could be if we made the effort. And good examples of how – to a greater or lesser extent – ageing is a matter of mental attitude.

The problem – with most of us – is simply a matter of *gradually* slowing down. This is not because our bodies, during our thirties and forties, necessarily dictate that we should, but because life for most of us has by then become settled around a regular family routine which simply has not been geared to give us regular exercise.

This is very bad news for us, although we do not feel the ill effects at once. Our bodies *need* physical exercise as much as they require food, and to give them (often an excess of) the second, while denying them the first, is clearly to invite the arrival of a whole range of ills we tend to associate with the middle years.

Certainly, many of us *are* naturally less vigorous after, say, thirty-five, than we were at twenty or twenty-five. But the worst attitude to take is one of resignation and passive acceptance, as exemplified by such expressions as 'Of course, I'm forty now, can't expect to run about as I *did when I was young*.' Or, 'I'm getting on for fifty – *you have to expect aches and pains when you reach my age!*'

Exercise slims you down whatever your age, by putting up the BMR (basal metabolic rate) – the rate at which you utilize food fuel at rest – and this increase continues for at least 24 hours *even after you have stopped exercising*. The proviso is that you keep up aerobic exercise for at least half an hour.

Aerobic exercise is the type that makes demands upon your heart and lungs, makes you breathe more quickly, makes you perspire, and makes your heart beat more rapidly. More important, it increases the rate at which you take in – and utilize – oxygen.

A short tear along the high street in pursuit of a disappearing bus, doesn't count – your leg muscles use up the oxygen already in them. Jogging for half an hour when you are only fit enough to jog for ten minutes is not aerobic exercise either (it could also be dangerous). You become intolerably breathless, and more oxygen is not being made use of, because your tissues and organs are not sufficiently fit to respire at the necessary rate.

Proper aerobic exercise is an individual issue. It is highly relevant to your present fitness state, and is defined as taking place when your pulse increases by a certain amount, according to your age and present pulse rate (16). It is also essential that the exercise be sustained for five to ten minutes, depending on your present fitness state.

With respect to how much extra energy this half hour of proper aerobic exercise uses up (and *do* work up to this time interval *gradually*) – according to Dr Newsholme, the Oxford biochemist responsible for this research (17), the answer is at least half as much again. The secret, he says, is that excess fat stores, rather than muscle and liver glycogen, are turned to as an energy source.

Just think what this means! Say you attend an aerobics class once a week for an hour, where you burn up 250 calories. Or you roller skate for an hour, and burn up 350. Whatever you do over the next 24 hours – even if you are asleep for eight or nine of them – you burn up an extra 125 in the first instance, or a further 175 in the second. That makes your aerobic workout worth 250 + 125 = 375 calories worth of energy expended (over and above your normal expenditure); or your roller skating hour worth 350 + 175 = 525 calories.

On the other hand, glycogen is utilized when we exercise vigorously for shorter spells of time. This may explain why a short sharp burst of exercise can leave you starving and not really affect your surplus fat. As soon as the glycogen has been used up, it has to be replaced, and we experience hunger. It takes thirty minutes or more to send your body into 'overdrive', and make use of unwanted fat layers.

2   No medical cause can be discovered for the preponderance of muscle aches and pains many menopausal women complain of. But this is what Donald Norfolk, a well-known osteopath, physical fitness adviser and author has to say about them (18):

The modern housewife suffers more 'fibrositic pain than her grandmother, even though her home is now equipped with every conceivable labour-saving gadget. The reason is that her daily routine deprives her of much opportunity to bend, twist, stretch and turn, while not sparing her the fatiguing postural strain of standing over sinks, work-tops and ironing-boards. In fact she is now more immobilized than ever before. For hours on end she stands and sits in positions of postural strain. Fibrositis, backache and degenerative arthritis . . . have strong causative links with our modern sedentary way of life.'

Fibrositis (muscular rheumatism), it seems, is caused by poor posture and tension, causing us to hold our back, trunk and neck muscles in anatomically unsuitable positions for long periods without relaxing. Proper exercise, however, whatever type we choose, causes the muscles to contract and relax alternately rather than to maintain a prolonged state of muscular contraction. This is healthy muscular action, as opposed to the type that imposes an injurious strain.

Backache is also due to poor posture and muscular tension, together with lack of exercise which weakens the back muscles and predisposes to obesity. This in turn places more postural strain on the spine, as does the development of weak abdominal, buttock and lumbar muscles – and makes active exercise even less attractive than it seemed before the chronic problems developed.

Exercise, however, reduces excess weight, corrects posture, strengthens muscles and relieves the hours of unremitting strain that helped cause backache in the first place.

Osteoarthritis is a degenerative disease of the joints, which many doctors attribute to wear and tear. Research suggests, however, that this widespread joint problem is neither an aspect of increasing age nor due to overuse of the joints concerned. It is caused by 'the damaging effect of immobility'. Freedom, by and large, from this joint disorder can be gained by exercise, regularly taken.

3 Many adults (and some children) are persistently tired. Women are particularly likely to suffer from fatigue at the time of the menopause, partly due to tension, anxiety, hot flushes and depression, all of which interfere with sleep patterns, and partly due to lack of stimulus.

Very few women realize when the second of these is true, and may protest that they are busy with jobs and housework, cooking and shopping, and that life is one long stimulus from morning to night.

According to Donald Norfolk, though, four out of every five patients suffering from chronic fatigue do so for 'purely functional reasons', i.e. it is their lifestyle that is to blame, and not some underlying disease process such as glandular dysfunction, heart disease or anaemia.

Mr Norfolk does not suggest aerobic exercise as a cure for all of life's ills. He presents the idea of what he terms a 'dynamogenic lifestyle', in which life is lived to full capacity, with gentle exercise and a steady pace of work playing as essential a role in the scheme as active, vigorous exercise, stimulating interests, adequate relaxation and an enjoyable, active sex life. This lifestyle as a whole, he says, is the best cure you can find for persistent tiredness.

4 It should be no news to anyone in our society nowadays that exercise prolongs life expectancy. Admittedly, this truth is not always expressed quite in this way. But when you think of some of the benefits regular exercise provides, it is little wonder that the link between active physical exertion and prolonged physical fitness is so strong.

Two elderly people who made a great impression on me when I was a child were engaged in horse riding and judo respectively. The first was a woman I used to see during my riding lessons in Hyde Park, where I used to spend Saturday mornings when pocket money permitted.

At the time I was struggling to master the mysteries of trotting in time to the horse's rhythm – in distinct preference to being joggled unceremoniously up and down like a sack of potatoes and losing one or both stirrups in the process. I asked my riding instructress who the fearless woman was whom we often saw, sweeping by on the back of her beautiful dapple grey and leaving an impressive cloud of dust behind her. I was told that she was Mrs D., well-known to all regular riders of Rotten Row, and 93 last birthday.

The second person to impress me with just how supple it is possible to be when you are elderly (and when you are twelve, seventy seems unimaginably ancient), was a judo master. I learned judo at the time at the Budokwai Club in Chelsea, and one afternoon went to a display of forward rolling breakfalls (and other solo tatami feats) by an acknowledged Japanese master and ninth dan (i.e. he had nine degrees of black belt!).

He held the room spellbound with his litheness, his physical subtlety, his breathtaking, perfect physical control and prowess. The teacher of our class asked us afterwards if any of us knew the master's age. He looked a youthful fifty, and he would have passed for forty-five with ease.

He was, we learned (I later confirmed this), fast approaching eighty.

It would, of course, be impossible for an eighty-year old (even a very fit one) to develop such physical powers from scratch, never having learned this type of exercise. The reason Mr W. was able to perform as he did, was because he had always been used to doing it, and he had quite simply never acquired the wish to stop.

Not for him the feeling that he'd reached forty and could expect rapid deterioration to set in forthwith!

Quite how does regular aerobic exercise maintain the body's youthful state? Apart from maintaining a normal body weight, and an attractive figure, exercise has the following rejuvenatory effects:

- It increases stamina (energy reserve and exercise tolerance) by increasing the amount of glucose (i.e. ready energy) stored as glycogen in the muscles, and by training the body's tissues to use oxygen to their maximum capacity.

  As we saw above, this helps to diminish stored fat and increase 'lean body mass' – the active, useful, skeletal muscular tissue under our voluntary control. But more than this, it improves our 'staying power' to the extent that more and more exertion can be made when required.

  Running upstairs, a quick sprint for a train, and cycling to the shops rather than driving there, become – and remain – part of your usual everyday activities.

- The chances of heart and circulatory disease developing are much reduced, in a number of ways. Firstly the heart beats more strongly and efficiently, and hence its workload of keeping the blood circulating is less fatiguing to it.

Secondly, it improves venous return (the return of vein blood) from the feet and legs, improving the rate of filling of the right atrium into which vein blood from the body drains. Improved passage of blood in the lower extremities upwards against the pull of gravity protects against the development of varicose veins, swollen ankles, varicose eczema and – at a later stage – the possible development of a varicose ulcer.

Thirdly, it improves the circulation of blood in the coronary arteries that supply the heart muscle, and which are the root of the problem when a heart attack (i.e. coronary thrombosis) occurs.

Fourthly, exercise reduces high blood pressure and tends to keep it at a normal level.

Fifthly, regular exercise raises the blood level of high density lipoproteins (HDLP are helpful blood fats), and reduces the blood levels of the harmful low density lipoprotein (LDLP) and cholesterol involved in arterial disease (atheroma).

5 The fact that regular exercise reduces stress, makes it especially beneficial during the menopause. We saw in an earlier chapter that menopausal symptoms are far more inclined to bother you if you are stressed, anxious and prone to worry over small details, than if you are calm, a non-worrier and live a busy, active life.

Two types of situation, in diametrical contrast to one another, are equally apt to produce tension, anxiety and depression around the time of the menopause. The first is when life becomes emptier than usual, a typical example being when the children leave home. You may have looked forward to this for years, longing for neatness and silence, and the opportunity to spend the days the way *you* would like to spend them. Now, suddenly, you miss them dreadfully, and find the days – not enlivened by new hobbies, fun trips to the shops, or visits to your friends – but dragging aimlessly past, while you fall prey to anxiety, depression and a host of minor health problems.

The second situation likely to cause problems is that of a busy, responsible job which you are more than capable of managing, but about which you suddenly start to feel anxious, unsure and tense. Your concentration – you feel – is not what it was, even a year ago. You know your boss is aware how old you are – and you also know that others would be pleased to step into your shoes.

To make matters worse, you find you can't even drink a cup of coffee without it bringing on a hot flush; and your nervous tension makes you snap at your secretary, colleagues and even your boss!

Before you seriously get sick with depression in the first situation, or resign from the second, do try exercise! Nothing could possibly seem less appealing at the moment – or less likely to help. But pent-up anxiety and unexpressed tension make for the development of neurotic illness, and it is better to deal sensibly with them now than suffer from full-blown anxiety attacks, phobias or actual physical illness later on.

The means by which a half-hour jog, a swim or a skipping session can help, is by providing an outlet for pent-up emotional energy. You may feel drained and exhausted rather than emotionally charged – but this in itself is a sign both that stress is your enemy, and that he's winning the battle.

Doubts and fears can come naturally at the 'change', especially with a change of lifestyle, and especially when your work is affected by symptoms you don't know how to deal with. The inner tensions and fears, and/or the stress of 'trying to keep up', trigger your primitive 'flight or fight' mechanism into pouring out an overflow of adrenalin from your adrenal glands.

You are primed for emergency action, perhaps your mouth goes dry, your skin feels prickly, your muscles are tense, your appetite negligible. Don't be surprised if your heart beat quickens, your pupils dilate or your hands tremble. All these are physical reactions to the hormone you are pouring into your bloodstream, and to which you are giving no other outlet.

The solution is to express pent-up energy generated by worry and anxiety in a form of exercise you enjoy. Nobody said you had to suffer to become fit, only that it will require a sustained effort. You can have no idea – until you have tried it – how immensely satisfying it is to smash all the anger and frustration you feel into the forward drive of a tennis or badminton racquet. Nor how justifiably pleased with yourself you feel, when you find, after persisting for a month, that you are beginning to feel more relaxed and self-confident.

For depression, exercise is one of the most effective drugless remedies in existence. You may have heard of a jogger's 'high' – the feeling of euphoria resulting from the release of hormone chemicals called endorphins during aerobic exercise. This is one of the many bonuses you gain, once you are able to exercise for long enough for it to happen.

But you do not have to wait, to have your spirits lifted by exercise. As soon as your pulse rate goes up, and you start to breathe more quickly – adrenalin is being released into your system in a healthy manner, and you feel livelier, more optimistic and far more capable of dealing with everyday affairs.

6 Not a great deal is known about *how* exercise improves your sex life. Its aphrodisiac effect has been attributed to the release of chronic anxiety and inner tension, general health improvement, greater vitality (as stamina and energy reserves improve, you have more zest for living), and an increased output of sex hormones.

My own feeling is that the improvement is due to a combination of all these factors. When you are menopausal, it is doubtful whether the flagging ovaries are capable of secreting more oestradiol than they are already. What could conceivably happen is that the improved blood circulation close to the fat layer results in an increase in the output of supplemental oestrogen.

It is within the fat layer below the skin, if you remember, that the 'extra' oestrogen supply is made. If my suggestion is correct, this would account, not only for the boost your sex drive receives from regular exercise, but also for the improvement in other menopausal problems.

With respect to *how* you should go about getting fit, I must emphasize the necessity of choosing something that you already enjoy doing, or which you are sure you would enjoy learning. The modern view of exercise is not the same as that of old-fashioned medicine – i.e. that it only does you good if it's nasty! Anyway, you'll be sure to give up something you hate or find boring.

Two good tips before we take a look at putting your re-introduction to exercise into practice. Firstly, try to find another beginner to exercise with – tell your husband it would do him the world of good, or ask a friend to join you. Alternatively, join a class – group workouts are fun.

If you have to exercise solo, don't do too much at first. Take aerobic exercise gently and have sympathy with your body which will do nothing but protest if you try to force it into a new life pattern without due preparation. Limber up for five minutes before you start a session, bending down low and stretching upwards, bobbing up and down on the balls of your feet and perhaps skipping with a rope.

You should also check your pulse rate after exercising, to make certain that you are not overdoing things (see below). You want the exercise session to do you good, not harm, and strained muscles and fatigue will do nothing to convince you that exercise is worthwhile.

Here is some advice based on excellent exercise for beginners tips published in *New Health* magazine, November 1983 issue.

In order to tell whether the exercise you have just taken was aerobic, check your pulse straight after exercising for five to ten minutes. Suppose you are forty-seven years old, and your pulse rate is between 105 and 140 after exercising for ten minutes. You will have achieved aerobic exercise by fulfilling two requirements.

Firstly your pulse will have risen to between 60 and 80% of the maximum rate for your age. Secondly, the effort will have been sustained for sufficiently long for it to count. (See Table 1.)

Table 1

Pulse rates for aerobic exercise – check your pulse after
exercising to find out if the exercise was aerobic

Age	Maximum pulse rate	60–80% of max. pulse rate
under 25	200	120 to 160
25–30	195	117 to 156
30–35	190	114 to 152
35–40	185	111 to 148
40–45	180	108 to 144
45–50	175	105 to 140
50–55	170	102 to 136
55–60	165	99 to 132
60–65	160	96 to 128
over 65	155	93 to 124

Jogging, swimming and cycling all offer the opportunity for
aerobic exercise, providing you follow the rules about pulse and
time duration.

New Health suggests a 'seven stages to fitness' regimen,
arranged both according to the days of the week, and according to
seven stages of achievement. You graduate from one to another as
and when you are ready to do so – advisers on the *New Health*
scheme suggest spending two to three weeks on each stage. When
you have reached stage five, your heart will have started to benefit
from the programme.

Table 2

Stage	Sat*	Sun†	Mon	Tues*	Wed	Thurs†	Fri	Total
1	10	–	–	5	–	5	–	20
2	15	–	–	5	–	10	–	30
3	20	–	–	10	–	10	–	40
4	25	10	–	10	–	15	–	60
5	30	15	–	15	–	20	–	80
6	35	15	–	25	–	25	–	100
7	40	20	–	30	–	30	–	120

The asterisked days indicate when you should exercise aerobically – and how long for. *New Health* suggest you pick jogging, but it's for you to choose.

The days marked with a dagger represent some activity such as walking, gardening or other aerobic exercise (you can easily make gardening or walking aerobic – just remember to check your pulse each time after ten minutes). The remainder are rest days.

Chapter Five

Overcome stress — and relax

We saw in Chapter Four that reaction to stress is basically the 'flight or fight' mechanism of early man. It is the physiological response to threat or danger, and stands us in extremely good stead when we *are* faced with a situation which requires total awareness and concentration, followed by lightning judgement and instant physical action.

Imagine that you are alone in the house, and are roused at four in the morning by the sound of a muffled rustle and a thump downstairs. You have no problem waking up! No alarm or cup of tea is necessary to set all your faculties on alert control. The next second probably sees you sitting bolt upright in bed, perspiring, with your heart hammering wildly, and your mouth dry.

However terrified you may be of burglars, the chances are that, if attacked, you could put up a good fight. At this very second, your mind is racing to decide where the nearest heavy weapon of defence might be. And since your blood is at this second being directed towards your arm and leg muscles, full of sugar and oxygen to prepare for action, you would in fact give a better account of yourself, if the occasion demanded, than you would ever give yourself credit for.

When you finally screw up your courage and tiptoe down the stairs, clutching a stiletto boot in one hand and an aerosol can of deodorant in the other — only to discover that the cat had been pulling a very dead chicken carcass through his cat door — the tension drains away. Instead of being charged for action, you now feel cold and trembly, maybe a little nauseous, and you want to go to the loo.

The adrenal glands react instantly to an emergency situation, by pouring out adrenalin into your bloodstream. What you are experiencing, when you go 'weak with relief', is the after-effects of this hormone which is, after all, one of the most powerful chemicals the human body manufactures.

The kind of frightening situation I have described is an ordeal at the time, but not in itself injurious. Had you actually found an intruder, you would have been very glad of your ability to react speedily and with precision. Other circumstances in which you may have been in debt to your adrenal glands include interviews, examinations, and road hazards encountered while driving.

Chattering teeth, wanting to pass water every five minutes and a thumping heart, are unpleasant – but the extra adrenalin secreted before you face a selection committee or an examination paper, actually helps you to give your best performance. And your ability to avoid a dog in the road, and at the same time miss a child who rushes out after a football, is also due to the co-ordination between your adrenal glands and your nervous system.

We even impose stress upon ourselves from choice. Many of us thrive on risk and danger, and the methods we as individuals use to obtain them are legion. They range from the obviously risky pursuits of hang-gliding, mountaineering and parachuting, through a whole spectrum of possibilities, to the equally perilous game of inciting a possessive partner to a jealous rage in which he might – just *might* – get violent.

Unsought forms of stress *are* harmful, however. There are two main types, both capable of causing serious physical and mental damage depending upon how we deal with them. The first type is the stressful life event. We have all experienced one or several of these at some time, and they range from breaking off an engagement, getting married, giving birth, and losing a parent or partner, to getting divorced, having an operation, your children leaving home, and going into hospital. The menopause is considered – unnecessarily, I suggest – to fit into this category.

The second type of stress consists of the constant stream of minor problems to which we are all subject. The arrival of bills weeks before the next cheque is due; a nagging husband; looking after demanding elderly parents, are common stresses. Noisy or nosy neighbours; queueing in crowded shops and supermarkets; driving round and round the block trying to find somewhere to park; and tearing through the week's shopping because in desperation you've had to park on double yellow lines, are others we've all experienced.

Have you noticed, though, how some people seem to cope with stressful situations so much better than others?

To be strictly accurate, none of these last mentioned 'stresses' is in fact the real source of the problem. They are experiences most of us would agree are trying. But *stress* really describes our reaction to them, not the events in themselves. None of them is capable of inflicting stress unless we co-operate and react accordingly. And this, in turn, depends upon our temperaments, our past experiences, our state of physical and mental health, and the habit patterns we learned from our parents.

This is why what amounts to a trivial annoyance to one person will cause anxiety, anger and a high degree of stress in another. We've seen the effects of adrenalin under genuine conditions demanding 'flight or fight'. Just think of the effects of shot after shot of 'emergency' adrenalin being pumped into the system scores of times every day. This is what happens to a person who reacts badly to stressful situations.

In order to cope with the situation, the body tries to adapt. The heart rate rises, the muscles remain tense, and the adrenal glands work overtime to provide extra adrenalin. The problem is that we were not intended to cope with a perpetually threatening environment, and the unnatural demands made upon us soon affect our health.

Instead of collapsing prematurely from physiological exhaustion, small warning signs appear that all is not well. We become tired and irritable, suffer from headaches, digestive upsets, and broken sleeping patterns; and complain of aches and pains for which no muscular or bone disorder can be found responsible.

If this is the stage we have reached at the time the menopause starts, it is not difficult to see the reason for the many physical and mental problems that can occur.

If we do nothing to reduce the stress factors that bombard us, and nothing about the way we let them affect us, then we should not be surprised if eventually we succumb to serious health problems. The number of disorders in which stress reactions are known to play a significant role grows yearly. At the present time it includes high blood pressure, strokes, coronary arterial disease, chronic muscular aches and pains, arthritis, cancer, peptic ulcers, hiatus hernia, migraine headaches, premature ageing, the premenstrual syndrome, chronic anxiety, depression and phobias.

The muscular rheumatism, hot flushes, anxiety attacks, lack of confidence, poor memory and concentration, fatigue, disturbed sleeping patterns and headaches associated with the menopause are also known for certain to be severely aggravated by tension.

That is why learning how to cope successfully with stress factors is a vital aspect of healthy living around the time of the 'change'. We have dealt with two important stress reducers so far – a wholefood diet and regular exercise. The next step is to learn a relaxation method, and to practise it daily. The ones I suggest as most appropriate are autogenic training, yoga and meditation, and autohypnosis. I also mention the benefits of biofeedback training as a useful adjunct to any of these methods.

1 Autogenic Training

The word 'autogenic' means 'generated from within'. Its aim is to enable the person practising it to combat his or her body's 'flight or fight' response to stress factors. It achieves this by gentle exercises in body awareness and relaxation, which bring about a state of mind called 'passive concentration'. Once you have mastered this technique – and it is not a difficult one to learn – you can 'switch on' the relaxed and tranquil state whenever necessary.

Autogenic training – 'autogenics' – is generally learned by person to person contact with a teacher, either privately or as part of a group. First the basic principles are taught, and you are asked to practise them two or three times daily. After that, it is sometimes possible to learn a special technique designed to help a specific problem.

This is how Miss A. M., a fifty-two year-old unmarried school teacher troubled with hot flushes, nervous tension and irritability, describes her experience of autogenics.

'I don't normally go in for that sort of thing – but I went to the first session on the advice of a friend who had found autogenics very helpful for her premenstrual tension.

'I had private instruction from a recommended teacher, since I wasn't able to go at the times the groups were held. I was a bit disappointed after the first lesson – it all seemed so absurdly simple, I couldn't imagine that it would do much for me.

'Anyway, I was told – and shown how – to sit really comfortably. I'd gone along in a straight skirt and blouse, nylons and high heels, straight from school, but my instructress – a lady about my age called Maria – recommended that I buy a track suit. She advised me to use it for practising and for future sessions as everyday clothes can be so restricting.

'I never thought I'd be buying modern gear at my time of life – but anyway, I took her advice and now I wouldn't be without it. There are three suitable positions in which to perform the exercises – sitting down, either on an upright chair or in an armchair, and lying down.

'Whichever you choose, say lying on a sofa as I do during the session, you start by stretching each limb and your back muscles, as much as you can without hurting yourself, then immediately let yourself go limp.

'If you've stretched really properly, you can feel the tension flowing out of your limp muscles – it's quite an art, getting all of yourself to relax at once. I had a bit of a problem with my neck and jaw muscles at first, but apparently that is very common.

Then, over the next few sessions (there were eight in all), I was shown how to enter a state of deep relaxation, by what is called visualization.

'I had to let every single bit of me go floppy and limp, and then breathe deeply and slowly, counting each breath. I had to concentrate on exactly how it felt when air entered my lungs, and how it felt when I breathed out.

'Once you are able to concentrate completely on this exercise, you find yourself becoming very calm and going sort of 'deep'. You could be roused, but you don't want to be — you are just perfectly happy concentrating on breathing in and out. This is the state of "passive concentration".

'I then had to imagine something about a part of my body — for instance, that my feet were warm, or that my legs were very heavy. I had to think about whatever it was, and repeat the fact to myself three times. It wasn't long before I started to experience whatever it was I was supposed to be feeling.

'Maria taught me right from the first, how to come out of this state and return to normal consciousness — that's very important. I first open my eyes, then I clench my fists and bring them up to touch my shoulders. Finally, I extend my arms as widely as I can, and yawn hugely!

'Between the weekly sessions, I kept to the advice I'd been given, and practised three times daily. I still do, in fact. It only takes about fifteen minutes, and I do it before leaving for school, during the lunch break and when I get home. During my last lesson, Maria said I could imagine my face growing cool, so that I could use this in future for my hot flushes.

'To tell you the truth, I'd already had a go at this at home and it had worked. Now I can avert hot flushes if ever I feel one coming on, simply by repeating to myself that my face is cool. But I get them very rarely nowadays anyway, since my level of tension has greatly lessened.

'I find I am far more relaxed than I have ever been — and if an especially naughty class does start to get the better of my patience, then I concentrate on my breathing for a few moments, and say the word "tranquillity" to myself, slowly, several times over.

'I am one hundred per cent better for autogenics, and I am not a bit tempted to ask my GP for hormone replacement therapy.'

It is important to mention that autogenics is not suitable for people with certain types of mental problem. It is possible, when in the state of passive concentration, to find that suppressed thoughts and memories, stored in the subconscious mind, rise to the surface, in a process known as abreaction. This can be very helpful, as it releases a lot of inner tension, but it could be unwise for some people – for instance, someone suffering from schizophrenia, or from manic-depression. If you are in any doubt, it is best to check with your GP or specialist, or with the autogenics teacher with whom you wish to learn.

The London Centre for Autogenic Training mentions a number of stress-related disorders for which autogenics has been found helpful. They include: 'Tiredness, insomnia, anxiety, examination nerves, circulatory problems including stress-related heart disorders, high blood pressure, migraine.'

Others – specially relevant to this book – are 'being overweight, nervous sweating, alcohol and tobacco problems, feelings of depression, inferiority, tension and hostility. Gynaecological problems, including premenstrual tension and menopausal symptoms, and dependence upon anti-depressants, tranquillizers, sleeping tablets, blood pressure drugs and other types of medication.'

2 Yoga and Meditation

Although yoga is known to have been practised in India for at least 6000 years, it was not until the 1960s that the majority of people in the West became acquainted with its practice. At first, its acceptance and growth so many thousands of miles from its country of origin may have seemed no more than another aspect of the hippy movement. Its critics tended to associate it with 'flower power', pot smoking, and bare-footed teenagers massing in support of the Beatles' friend and guru, the Maharishi Mahesh Yogi.

But the benefits of yoga so quickly became apparent that its transplantation to a new culture succeeded, albeit with a number of modifications which have helped Westerners adapt to both its philosophical and its practical sides. Just as khaftans, leather thong sandals and incense sticks are unremarkable features nowadays in any English market, so yoga is a familiar choice on the subject list of many evening class groups throughout the country.

Yoga is also being studied scientifically all over the world (19). At the IC Yogic Health Centres in Lonavla and Bombay, India, detailed records are kept of patients treated for chest complaints, digestive disorders, obesity and diabetes. Doctors at The Third Clinic of Medicine, Krakow, Poland, have examined the effects of yoga posture on the composition and quality of the blood. (During the headstand pose, patients were found to inhale 10% less oxygen, resulting in 33% more oxygen being used by the blood.)

At the Veterans' Administration Hospital in Sepulveda, California, Dr Barbara Brown, researching the brain waves of regular yoga practitioners, commented: 'Eventually, most diseases may be treated by establishing healthful brain wave patterns, either by self-training or by mechanical means.'

A basic principle of yoga is that good health consists of the harmonious integration of body, mind and spirit. This is also the basic tenet of holistic medicine and the truth of this simple fact is becoming more and more apparent to us as we learn more about the power of the mind – and of the spirit – to influence our lives for good or ill.

This is what Professor Henry Sigerist, of the Department of the History of Medicine, John Hopkins University, had to say in 1961, when he challenged the orthodox conviction that the mind played little part in healing. In the second volume of his history of medicine, he stated: 'Every cell of our organism is controlled by the nervous system which conveys impulses of the mind.'

Since the will to get better is in so many cases a decisive healing factor – 'how much more potent must be the effect of a mind concentrated in meditation. We may think of autosuggestion, autohypnosis; but whatever the mechanism may be, there can be no doubt that a philosophy such as that of Yoga has great medical potentialities.'

There are a number of different kinds of yogic practice, some concentrating upon a limited number of postures (asanas) and the control of breathing, some – at the opposite end of the spectrum – attaching great importance to philosophy and meditation. The type known as Hatha yoga is the sort most of us are familiar with. This aims at correcting the student's posture, and establishing the principles of proper breathing. In this way, the overall health of the body, mind and spirit improve since greater harmony is established between all three of them.

The most outstanding benefit of yoga is the lessening of inner tension, and the improvement in the way we react to daily stresses. This is why so many stress-induced or stress-aggravated conditions disappear or greatly improve in response to daily yoga sessions.

This is what Mrs B. L., a forty-seven year-old mother of two teenage sons, has to say about yoga.

'I practise it at least four times a week – every day, when I get the chance. I was never very good at disciplining myself, before I took up yoga – in particular, I used to "binge eat" around the time of my periods, and even more so when the "change" started. But once I discovered what yoga could do for my muscular aches and pains, depressions, night sweats and hot flushes, I didn't need to persuade myself to practise it! In fact, right from the start I looked forward to that daily half hour of peace and quiet.

'I started going to classes once a week with my friend, when I read a magazine article about how yoga can help women overcome health problems. We were taught three simple postures the first week, as well as the Corpse posture, which consists of lying perfectly still on the floor with your hand and arms by your sides and ankles apart. We always begin and end a session with the Corpse – it stills the mind at the start, and gets you to relax after a busy day.

'Doing it again at the end, our teacher told us, sort of lets all the benefit of the session sink right into your system, so that you carry the relaxed feeling away with you.

'We learned to do all the postures slowly, and to remain aware of our breathing as we carried them out. We had to breathe slowly and deeply throughout the session, and we were reminded of the benefits of deep breathing whenever we were faced with stressful situations outside.

'We learned about three new postures a session, and had individual help with breathing and posture problems. Mr Miller (our teacher) also used to check that we were fully relaxed during the Corpse posture that ended the session.

'We particularly liked the three lessons in meditation that came as an optional extra at the end of the twelve-week yoga course. My friend's blood pressure has gone down since we started meditating, and we both find it comes quite naturally to meditate for a few minutes straight after doing our yoga, or during one of the postures.

'There are lots of different ways of meditating, but what Mr Miller taught us suits both my friend Jean and myself. You sit in a comfortable chair – not straight after a meal, or alcohol – after you've taken the phone off the hook and made sure you're unlikely to be disturbed. You look at something both non-distracting and beautiful – I always choose a dark green glass vase, which picks up the light from the standard lamp behind my chair.

'Then you say what is called your "mantra" over to yourself, letting the syllables linger in your mind, and filling your mind with their sound so that all ordinary thought disappears. Jean sets an alarm, but I just come out of it naturally after fifteen minutes or so. My breathing gets quiet and still and I feel wonderful when I stop!

'I've lost nearly a stone in six months since I took up yoga. Not because it actually slims you, but I'm so much less tense that I no longer eat bars of chocolate between meals. And yes, my menopausal symptoms have all but disappeared. I got a hot flush about a month ago, when the car ahead of me in a traffic jam went into reverse and backed into my husband's new Mini, breaking a head lamp! But under everyday conditions I feel fine and my husband's getting interested in taking up yoga too – he says I am so much easier to live with!'

3 Autohypnosis

Perhaps of all the techniques we are looking at here, autohypnosis may seem the most strange. This may be because hypnotism itself still retains – to a certain extent – the image of a weird, unorthodox, even dangerous practice. It could also be because hypnosis, in one form or another, is nowadays associated in many people's minds with cults such as the Moonies, who are said by some to utilize hypnotism to control the willpower of their disciples.

In fact, the origins of hypnotism were established before the days of recorded history, for healing in a trance state is one of the most ancient of the medical arts. It worked for the ancient Egyptians and the early Greeks and the Persians, in the same way as it works nowadays, by tapping the power of the subconscious mind. And although – like all forms of therapy – it can be used, under certain conditions, to do harm, there is nothing but good to be said of its use in the treatment of stress reactions and unwanted symptoms.

'Tapping the power of the subconscious mind' is not as difficult – nor as vague – an undertaking as it sounds. The subconscious region of the mind is the store house of every single one of our past memories – and this includes the sum total of every experience, pleasant and unpleasant, minor and momentous, which we have ever had.

The conscious area, on the other hand, is the 'awareness' faculty with which we relate to our environment, i.e. with which we perceive, understand, decide, and initiate actions. This represents only the 'tip of the iceberg' in comparison with the subconscious region, which accounts in all for about nine tenths of our total mind power.

As well as being our memory store, the subconscious mind plays another vital role in our lives. It helps to regulate our autonomic nervous system, and by so doing, is one of the factors that control our heart beat, our glandular secretions, our rate of breathing, blood pressure and digestive functions. If you add to this information the fact that the subconscious mind will act upon any direction it receives, so long as that direction does not conflict with the basic beliefs of the person concerned, you will begin to see the reason why the subconscious mind has such an important role to play in health and disease.

There are a number of ways of getting a message through to the subconscious mind. Hypnotherapists do this by distracting the conscious awareness. This used to be done by getting you to focus on a pendant on a swinging chain, or on a small light. Nowadays, it is more likely to be by asking you to count backwards from, say three hundred to one, while the therapist places his finger on your forehead and asks you to roll your eyes upwards in an effort to 'see' the point he is touching.

Meanwhile, he suggests over and over in a monotonous voice that you are getting drowsy, tranquil and relaxed and, after a few minutes, you have entered a state of light trance. He can then communicate directly with your subconscious mind, making whatever suggestions are required for your benefit.

Autohypnosis works by inducing a similar state of light trance in yourself, and then suggesting to yourself whatever you need to suggest. If you wish to lose, say, tension, irritability and aggressive feelings, and remain calm when bombarded by stress, then you would suggest these in a positive way, each time you used the technique. Let Mrs C. S., a fifty-three-year-old, widowed accounts clerk, give an account of her experience with autohypnosis.

'I learned autohypnosis from a book, but some people go to hypnotherapists to learn, and this is probably easier in the long run. My reason for learning the technique was the fact that I'd heard a radio programme about it, and wanted something to help me with my menopausal symptoms.

'When I started autohypnosis, I had been widowed for fifteen months. My periods had begun to grow scanty while my husband was alive, but a month or so after he died, they stopped altogether and I started to get the most awful hot flushes. As you can see, I normally have a pale complexion, so a blushing attack – together with heavy perspiration – was terribly embarrassing. To add to it, I started bursting into tears for the slightest thing, my memory and concentration went to pieces, and I was afraid I'd lose my job. You can't afford to make mistakes when you're dealing with rows of figures – even if they are all computerized nowadays.

'Anyway, I will summarize how I use autohypnosis. First of all I choose a relaxed time of day – generally after I've got home from work and have had a bath and changed. Then I settle down in a comfortable armchair, in a dimly lit room, and gaze at a candle flame – an easy image to conjure up under other conditions, by the way, and also one that symbolizes peace and tranquillity to me.

'I then count backwards from ten to one, telling myself in my mind that as I descend the order of numbers, I get more and more relaxed, and deeper and deeper into a trance state. When I am ready, I "see" my face in my mind's eye, keeping cool, pale and unflushed, even when surrounded by stresses and worries, and repeat to myself, "I am cool and calm." I also say: "My memory is getting better and better", and "I feel happy, serene and relaxed." I do take the phone off the hook, as I try not to be disturbed – but I can easily rouse myself if someone comes to the door, or if something demands my immediate attention.

'Normally of course this does not happen – and I just come out of my nice, relaxed trance when I think I will, by counting back up to ten again from one, and picturing myself surfacing again from the trance state.

'At first I carried out a fifteen-minute trance session every evening – now I do it twice a week, and intend to continue with it as I feel the benefit in so many ways.

'If I feel I am getting a bit het up, I just picture my candle flame, and the feeling of relaxation comes over me.

'Actually, my memory *is* better now (it's six months since I started). It didn't improve for the first three months but, do you know, it didn't bother me! I very rarely get het up these days, and I certainly never burst into tears at work!

'My hot flushes were the first problem to improve, and I don't think I've had three in as many months. I am also coming to terms a little more with Wilfred's death – and I've bought a dog as company, something Wilf always asked me to do, should he be the first to go.'

Biofeedback

You may not have heard of biofeedback. The essential principle underlying it – that physiological changes accompany emotional changes – was first reported in the nineteenth century by scientists investigating hypnosis. More specifically, the French neurologist Charles Fere showed that variations in mood are accompanied by variations in the resistance of the skin to a small electric current.

Not a great deal of practical use was made of this discovery, however, apart from the invention of lie detectors, until the 1960s, when the potential of biofeedback for the treatment and prevention of illness was realized by several scientists in the USA.

One of these, Kamiya, a Chicago neuropsychiatrist, suggested that, since physical conditions are related to brain wave activity, it might be possible to alter the physical state by tuning in to a different wave length. Experiments involving students soon proved that this was possible. The group Kamiya worked with, for instance, were able to guess, each time a bell rang, whether they were producing the equivalent of long, medium or short brain waves. And they learned to produce waves of a different variety at will.

The relevance of all this today is that by combining the use of a biofeedback machine – which you can be trained to use – with Hatha yoga or autogenics, you can teach yourself, say, to cool one side of your face and not the other, or raise the temperature of one hand by several degrees.

These may seem pretty pointless exercises, but the obvious corollary is that the technique – or rather the combination of two techniques – can be applied to whatever is your special need.

If, for instance, you need to be able to 'turn off' a hot flush the moment you feel one is about to start, autogenics plus biofeedback can help you achieve this more rapidly than you would by using autogenics alone.

If, on the other hand, your main problem is tension and stress-related disorders – remember, a fair number of so-called menopausal symptoms cannot be traced to a low level of blood oestrogen and are believed to be stress-generated – then autogenics, or yoga, plus biofeedback will help you to overcome the problem.

Biofeedback is not a therapy, but is used either as a teaching aid to help you control your blood pressure, palpitations, migraine attacks, or hot flushes, or as a therapy adjunct, to help you put more into – and gain more benefit from – whichever therapy you have chosen.

The two chief biological data sources tapped to provide you with the parameters you require, are electrical skin resistance and brain waves. The information can be provided in a variety of forms – a tone that varies with mood is one, and the rise and fall of a needle along a graduated scale is another. Electrodes may be strapped to your scalp, or to the palms of your hands.

The particular method is immaterial. What is significant is the use you make of the information you receive, to gain as much control as possible over your interacting body, mind and spirit.

Chapter Six

Supplementary benefits

After writing as I have in Chapter Three about the benefits of wholefood eating, it will probably come as a surprise to you that I am an advocate of dietary supplements as well. How can you possibly need them, you may well wonder, if you eat plentiful supplies of whole grains, fruit, vegetables, sprouting seeds and nuts, and shun all the once-tempting junk food you used to eat?

If you already eat wholefoods – or are in the process of changing to them – then your diet is as healthy as you can possibly make it, practically speaking. All the same, it is likely – in one or two respects – to fall a little short of ideal. To eat a perfect diet you would have to grow all your own fruit and vegetables organically, know precisely what nutrients were in your soil, and also be certain of the origin of all the organic gardening aids you use.

In addition, you would have to be sure that all the eggs you eat were free range – from hens that never pecked up anything chemically undesirable in their free ranging farmyard. You would have to know that the fish you included in your diet had not swum into areas of sea or river containing radioactive or toxic waste material. And you would have to be equally sure that if you ever did touch red meat, the animals from which it came had never been given antibiotics, steroid injections or hormone treatment.

In addition to these requirements, it would be essential for you to live in a remote rural area far away from any source of industrial or environmental pollution; and you would also have to be quite sure that the atmosphere contained no traces of radio-active substances with which you might be bombarded.

Needless to say, you would also have to live a life free from harmful stress factors, including in your lifestyle only those helpful, challenging stresses that bring a gleam of excitement to the eye and a rush of exhilaration within.

You are probably thinking by now that the only light in the eye of anyone who could live according to such impossibly high principles would be the light of fanaticism. The requirements do constitute a very tall order indeed; and while there are people with the interest, time and money to attain such high standards – at least with respect to diet – they are a practical impossibility for most of us. The village stores, or the nearest supermarket, are the only choices we have and, with the limited time available, selecting the best food possible during our weekly shopping expedition is the best we can hope to manage.

Dietary supplements are therefore necessary to combat the possibly harmful effects of the 'hidden' threats in our food and environment. These include the pesticide sprays and inorganic fertilizers with which even 'organic' fruit and vegetables may have come into contact. And they are needed to combat the possibly carcinogenic effects of toxic waste in sea and river water – and therefore in fish.

They are needed to compensate for any vitamin, mineral or essential fatty acid deficiency we may suffer, due to imperfect food products, the effects of stress, or both. And they are needed to give us certain definable advantages which medical research has revealed as available to us, now that more is known about human biochemistry and its requirements.

Just two of the many supplements from which we can benefit illustrate this point admirably. The first is evening primrose oil (Efamol) which supplies gamma linolenic acid (GLA). We need this in order to make hormone-like substances called prostaglandins of a type known as E1. (There are injurious prostaglandins you may have heard about in connection with disorders such as rheumatoid arthritis. E1 prostaglandins, however, are 'good' ones that are needed by all our body cells in the regulation of their moment by moment functioning.)

Under ideal conditions, we are able to manufacture all the GLA we require, and convert it into a chemical which in turn gets changed into the end product – E1 prostaglandins. We normally take in plenty of the starter material, linoleic acid, in the food we eat, as this is present in vegetable oils, margarine, and a number of plant products. What happens, though, is that many of us find the first stage of the chain – converting dietary linoleic acid into GLA – impossible, because the enzyme (organic catalyst) necessary for the conversion gets put out of commission by a variety of factors. These are too numerous to mention here in full, but the most interesting in the context of diet, lifestyle and the menopause include the effects of stress (too much adrenalin again), any artificial food additives with which we may come into contact, the effects of ageing and any animal (saturated) fats we may include in our diets.

No (or defective) conversion of linoleic acid into GLA means, of course, a deficient supply of the prostaglandin E1 end product. This affects a very wide range of bodily functions including weight gain, cholesterol level, mood, arthritic conditions, the reactions of our bodily cells to the hormones we produce, and the condition of our skin, nails and hair. Reactions to hormones include the premenstrual syndrome (PMS – often particularly troublesome in the premenopausal woman). Moods affected by low levels of prostaglandin E1 include depression (probably), and the emotional highs and lows common during PMS monthly phases.

Taking evening primrose oil (Efamol) supplies us with ready-made GLA, thus overcoming our conversion problem with linoleic acid. Our cells are quite capable then of converting GLA into the next stage of the process (called dihomo-gamma-linoleic acid), and thence into the vital prostaglandins.

The second case in point is eicosapentaenoic acid (EPA) which many people now take as the supplement MaxEPA. This is made by the Seven Seas company, famous for many years for their cod liver oil supplements, and now manufacturing a product that is proving to be of vital importance in man's fight against heart and arterial disease.

EPA is needed for the production of the prostaglandins – three series which control blood clotting and arterial spasm. EPA also improves the viscosity of the blood, and lowers both triglycerides and cholesterol (especially the type bound to low density lipoproteins now known to be linked with an increased incidence of heart disease).

EPA is known to be one of the key factors explaining the very low incidence of heart disease among the Eskimos compared with us in the West. The Japanese have a lower coronary rate, too, and the one striking factor common to the Japanese and the Eskimos, which is lacking in Westerners, is their high consumption of cold water oily fish such as cod, mackerel and herrings.

Research into the link between the consumption of deep sea fish and the reduced incidence of heart disease revealed that a 'key fatty acid, EPA, dramatically inhibits the formation of blood clots'. EPA is also effective in reducing the pain and swelling of rheumatoid arthritis.

The supplement MaxEPA was developed to enable anyone who did not want to eat oily fish every day to benefit from the effects of EPA. Many people take it for the protection it offers against heart disease, and for its second component fatty acid – DHA – (docosahexaenoic acid), a major constituent of the brain and the retina (20).

There are two other very good reasons why people take supplements regularly. One is in order to achieve the greatest degree of fitness possible, and the other is to combat the effects of drugs, many of which can induce vitamin deficiencies.

Super Fitness

We have seen in past chapters how the body and the mind can interact as a result of stress to produce a number of disorders, in particular those afflicting many women around the time of the menopause. So miserable can menopausal symptoms make you, in fact, that you may well feel that you would thankfully opt just for release from weight gain, hot flushes, a sore vagina and irritability, and be quite content with that, never mind some high flung notion of 'super fitness'.

Now I quite understand how you can come to hold that opinion, and I have discussed this point with many menopausal women when we have approached the topic of diet, lifestyle and supplements. However, I must emphasize that once you have achieved super fitness you will wonder why you ever put up with an inferior level of health. And the right supplements are essential in reaching this peak of vitality.

In sketching out the daily supplement requirements most suited to your needs, I must point out that 'needs' are an individual issue. The majority of women approaching or experiencing the menopause find that the plan suggested here suits them extremely well. If, however, you take the supplements I suggest, based on those worked out by the famous naturopath and author Leon Chaitow, and still feel that something is lacking, then the supplements only go part of the way to doing what they should for you. Your best course of action then is to consult a naturopathic practitioner/ nutritional expert and discuss with him/her your health history, lifestyle and diet and let them sort out what dietary supplements you need.

By far the most important supplements are the vitamins and minerals. Vitamins are naturally occurring chemical substances vital to life. In the main, we rely on our diet to supply us with all the vitamins we need, although we are capable of manufacturing one or two of them ourselves. Vitamins control the functioning of our body cells through enzymes, keeping them up to par, and able to carry out their complex activities of nutrient absorption and utilization as efficiently as they should.

The following vitamins have so far been named – without doubt more await discovery by scientists researching the mysteries of human nutrition: A (retinol, carotene); B complex group = B1 (thiamine), B2 (riboflavin), B3 (niacin), B5 (pantothenic acid), B6 (pyridoxine), B10 and B11 (growth factors), B12 (cyanocobalamin), B13 (orotic acid), B15 (pangamic acid), B17 (amygdalin), PABA (para-amino benzoic acid); choline; inositol. Vitamin C (ascorbic acid); D (calciferol, viosterol, ergosterol); E (tocopherol); F (essential fatty acids, also called EFAs); H (biotin); K (menadione); L (for lactation); M (folic acid); P (bioflavonoids); T (growth promoting substances); U (extracted from cabbage juice).

Minerals are minute quantities of certain elements needed for cellular function, and to enable vitamin activity to take place. Most of them are metals – e.g. calcium, chromium, cobalt, copper, iron, magnesium, manganese, molybdenum, potassium, selenium, sodium, vanadium and zinc. Others are non-metals – chlorine, fluorine, iodine, phosphorus and sulphur.

Generally speaking, vitamins are obtained commercially by extracting them from natural substances, rather than by synthesis in a laboratory. Vitamin A, for example, is derived from fish liver oil, and the best kind of vitamin C from rose hips.

Synthetic vitamins and minerals are less satisfactory than their naturally occurring counterparts, although there may be no difference between them when they are analysed. The synthetic forms are also capable of causing allergic reactions and gastrointestinal upsets, and these are far less likely to occur with the naturally occurring forms.

Three terms you will come across in connection with dietary supplements are 'chelation', 'time release' and 'fillers and binders'. These need explanation if you are new to dietary supplements. Firstly chelation (pronounced kee-lation) is the chemical process minerals have to undergo in our digestive systems before they can be adequately used. Once chelates have been formed, of calcium, for example, or of iron, the body can go ahead and put the mineral to the use for which it requires it. When natural chelation is defective, though, the particular mineral or minerals affected pass out of our bodies without having been of benefit to them.

We have now learned how to chelate minerals beforehand, and the point of buying them in their chelated state is so that we can use them to optimum effect. They are assimilated by the body between three and ten times more efficiently than their non-chelated equivalents.

Time release vitamins are ones that have been prepared in such a manner that they are released into our systems gradually, over a period of eight to twelve hours, rather than all at once. The advantage of this is that the level in the blood of whatever we are taking rises slowly and stays more or less constant for a considerable time, rather than reaching a peak briefly, and then being broken down and excreted by the kidneys.

Fillers and binders are the inert substances added to the active ingredient of a tablet or capsule to increase their bulk to manageable proportions and to bind the granules together so that they can be compressed into shape. Look carefully at the label of whatever you are buying – just as you would scrutinize the ingredients list of, say, a commercially prepared wholemeal loaf to discover what you were getting besides wholemeal flour, yeast and salt.

Besides filling and binding substances, there are other similar factors which may creep in to supplements of any type, including colouring matter, drying agents, disintegrators, flavourings and lubricants. Just make certain that you pick supplements that guarantee their whole contents to be naturally occurring, and devoid of synthetic additives. There is no point in taking supplements in order to combat the effects of stress (and that includes the chemical insults our systems receive many times a day if we eat commercially prepared food), if those supplements also contain artificial colouring matter and similar potentially harmful chemicals!

Here, then, is the supplement programme based on the Leon Chaitow regimen which I suggest is most helpful to women at the time of the menopause.

(i) High potency multiple vitamin and mineral (preferably time release), one morning and evening. Make sure that this supplement contains adequate vitamin D, which like calcium is essential to your campaign against osteoporosis. You should be getting 400 iu twice daily.

(ii) Six to ten brewer's yeast tablets daily, taken throughout the day at mealtimes.

(iii) Kelp tablets – one morning and evening.

(iv) MaxEPA – the recommended dose for maximum effect is five capsules twice daily, but if this seems a lot, eat as much oily fish as you can and reduce the dose by half.

(v) Garlic capsules – one morning and evening.

(vi) Calcium gluconate – 500 mg twice daily, if you eat a fair amount of foods containing calcium; 750 mg twice daily if you take in little in your diet.

Good sources of calcium include milk and milk products (go for the low fat variety), sardines, soya beans, salmon (eat the little bit of soft bone in the middle of tinned salmon as well as the flesh – it's extra calcium and delicious!). Also high in calcium are peanuts, walnuts, sunflower seeds, dried beans and green vegetables.

By the way, it is important to make sure that the amount of phosphorus you take as a supplement is half that of the calcium you include.

The above supplements, taken as part of a health regimen which includes a wholefood diet, exercise, relaxation and the other advice I have so far given, should clear up the majority of minor symptoms such as headaches, irritability and tiredness. It should also go a long way to protecting you from osteoporosis.

Hot flushes can be treated as follows:

(vii) Vitamin E, 400 iu, morning and evening. Some vitamin E supplements contain selenium – if yours does, make certain that it is in a dose of 50 mcg (micrograms) minimum. If it does not, take selenium as a separate supplement (not more than 100 mcg daily).

(viii) Vitamin C together with bioflavonoids, one gram morning and evening.

(ix) Stress B complex, in which the strength of the chief B vitamins is 50 to 100 mg.

The stress B complex tablets should help a great deal with poor ability to withstand stress, and I would advise you to take them even if you *think* you withstand stress pretty well, in either of the following circumstances: (a) if you have experienced a major stressful life event recently (see Chapter Five), or (b) if you think that the stress rating of your usual lifestyle is very probably high in comparison with that of other women of your age.

Also helpful in combating stress is the addition of the following supplements:

(x) Calcium pantothenate – 500 mg daily.

(xi) Efamol (oil of the evening primrose flower) – excellent for stress and to assist cellular metabolism in general (see above) – take at least one capsule morning and evening. Efamol is so beneficial (it is also believed to be a potent factor in combating the ageing process) that the maximum dose may be taken if you wish, and can afford it: five 500 mg capsules morning and evening.

NB The maximum dose is simply the largest dose that it has so far been found necessary by some people to take, in order to achieve maximum effect. There is no 'upper limit' to the amount of Efamol you can take from the safety point of view since – unlike drugs – it is entirely without toxicity.

This list may be ample for you to start off with, especially if you are not used to taking any supplements at all. If you want to pare your list down to the barest essentials I would suggest that you take a multivitamin and mineral tablet/capsule twice daily, an Efamol capsule twice daily, 400 iu vitamin E daily and your calcium supplement as above.

Here is a brief summary of what you can expect the various supplements I have recommended to do for you.

Multivitamin and mineral complex will supply the essential vitamins and minerals you need, and remove the uncertainty as to whether you are getting enough of everything, every day, from your diet. As we saw above, vitamins and minerals have a wide range of functions in the human body, and are vital to the overall control of metabolic processes.

Brewer's yeast (do not take this if you suffer from thrush). This yeast is one of the richest sources of organic iron, and provides good protein and the natural B complex vitamins (therefore being a stress fighter). It also supplies minerals, trace minerals (minerals we require in extremely small quantities such as selenium), and amino acids (the chemical units from which protein molecules are built).

Kelp is a type of seaweed and contains more vitamins and minerals than any other food. It is especially valuable as a source of B_2, niacin, choline, carotene and iodine, and has a normalizing effect on the thyroid gland, one of the main factors in controlling metabolic weight. If you are overweight, kelp is said to be able to help you to lose weight more easily, and if you are trying to gain more pounds, kelp is equally able to help you put weight on.

MaxEPA. This has been dealt with above.

Garlic. Besides supplying potassium (which is good for the heart and other muscles), vitamins B and C, calcium and phosphorus, garlic helps to lower the blood pressure, has natural antibiotic properties (not the type that encourage the growth of thrush), and helps to lower an abnormally raised blood pressure.

Calcium gluconate. This supplies most of the extra calcium you need to remain free from any appreciable degree of osteoporosis. Besides strengthening your bones (and your teeth), it helps to keep your heart healthy, enables you to make maximum use of iron, is useful to your nervous system, especially in the transmission of nerve impulses, and helps to rectify sleeping problems.

Vitamin E. This has many activities in the human body. Its special value to anyone going through the menopause is its effect upon hot flushes. Since vitamin E is a natural substance and not a drug, do not expect overnight results. It may take weeks or months to produce its full curative effects, but be patient because they are worth waiting for. Vitamin E also retards cellular ageing, increases your physical stamina, fights fatigue, prevents blood clots, and helps to keep your veins healthy and non-varicose. Both it and selenium help to combat the effects of inhaled pollutants, which tend to create what are known as free radicals, the formation of which is harmful to our cells.

Vitamin C is another antioxidant, i.e. like vitamin E it helps to protect us from free radical formation. It also fights bacterial infections, subdues allergic reactions, and decreases the incidence of cancer by 75% if taken in doses of between 1 and 10 grams daily, according to the vitamin C expert Doctor Linus Pauling.

Stress B complex. All the components of the B complex offer slightly different benefits, but collectively and in a sufficiently high dose they are a potent anti-stress aid.

Calcium pantothenate. This supplement aids in the building of antibodies, prevents fatigue and buffers you against the effects of stress. It also reduces the adverse effects of many antibiotics.

Chapter Seven

Sex can be better than ever

Whoever heard of sex getting *better* at and after the menopause? Certainly some women – like Mrs E. O. in Chapter One – claim that they find that it does. But couldn't many such claims be empty boasts, stemming – as did Mrs E. O.'s – from a mixture of self-doubt and compulsive wishful thinking?

There are so many varying attitudes to sex and sexuality at any given moment that there is little point in trying to sort through them here. The only aim of such an exercise would be to discover whether it is usually the woman who is to 'blame' for the sexual problems that characteristically arise between couples in their fifties. My own feeling is that it is safer and also closer to the truth, to steer clear of the word 'blame' altogether, and examine some of the actual problems that arise with a view to trying to solve them.

There is a widespread belief that women 'go off' sex when they go through the 'change'. Certainly – since the women I quoted in the first chapter were fairly representative of menopausal patients – a number do use it as an excuse not to make love any more. But, as was evident in these four cases, there is often much more behind sexual reluctance than a straightforward loss of libido. More frequently it is caused by physical discomfort, a lack of self-confidence and repressed feelings of aggression and fear.

You will notice that I said the four women we discussed earlier were representative of 'menopausal patients', not necessarily of menopausal women in general. Some do genuinely find that love-making remains just as exciting, and sometimes even improves, during the menopause.

These women may be looked upon as 'lucky' – but they do not possess some secret that no one else can share. Neither do they pay vast sums of money for rare aphrodisiacs or rejuvenation injections. All it takes to continue enjoying sex through and well beyond the menopause is a loving and considerate partner and a little practical know-how.

Before we look at the three specific problem spots I have referred to, here are a few words of advice about love-making in general. Firstly, please believe that the change of life *can* herald a change for the better in bed. The menopause *does* mean the end of having babies, but it also means no more contraception, period pains, premenstrual syndrome (PMS) – or 'off' days when sex is inconvenient.

If, for a number of reasons, sex has never been a bright spot in your marriage, think honestly about why this is so. If you have been unhappily married for years, but have stayed together for the sake of the children or out of long-established habit – now is the time to reconsider the situation. Now that the children are older and about to leave home to make their own lives, think hard about whether you really want yours to go on as it has for the past couple of decades.

You owe it to yourself to pluck up courage, and have an honest talk with your husband/lover, and decide what is best for both of you – even if that means the pair of you parting. You may feel afraid of going solo when you have already reached a half century in birthdays. But thousands of women who have tried it can attest that life is far more satisfactory when one is doing one's own thing – whatever one's age – than living a colourless half-life through fear of change.

On the other hand, let us suppose that although neither of you has really found much pleasure in sex, you are happy together and content to leave it that way. If this is really the case, then it is absolutely your privilege to do so and it would be an impertinence to offer you advice. However, it *could* just be that you might both find joy in sexual sharing at this time in your lives, if one of you (*you*!) were brave enough to broach the subject, and share your thoughts, problems and perhaps even fantasies (see below) with your partner.

The other possibility is that you and your husband or lover have had a good life together, and have found sex enjoyable. Now, suddenly, you don't want to be bothered with it, and this worries both of you and leads to rows. Rather than letting things deteriorate any further, consider whether any or all of the three factors discussed below apply to you. And have some sexual therapy as well to tide you over until you start to feel the benefit of some suggested changes. Sex therapy, by the way, can be very helpful to many couples with sexual difficulties. Most people – especially men – shy away from the thought of it, fearing that it would be embarrassing, brash and based on winkling out stories of one's failures in bed for the edification of a roomful of social workers. So far from the truth is this idea that I have encouraged many sensitive, even reluctant couples to make appointments with sex therapists, confident that they would be pleased with the outcome.

All but two, in fact, of a total of twenty-three couples, whose problems ranged from the commonplace to the bizarre, benefited a great deal from their therapy sessions. Therapy, incidentally, comprises private discussion of each partner alone with the therapist and perhaps a trainee therapist, followed by sessions involving both partners together.

There is no 'practical' side to the therapy, within the confines of the clinic. The accent is on relaxation and privacy, and the exercises the couple are advised to do are carried out at home with plenty of useful advice about making the experience as enjoyable as possible. Many women have told me that they have found it *less* embarrassing to talk about marital sexual problems in front of a therapist than it would be alone with their husbands at home. Men, too, have confided to me that, far from being made to feel either brutish or incompetent because they have 'failed' in some way to satisfy their wives or girlfriends, they have been impressed by their therapist's wisdom and skill in handling highly sensitive subjects in a down-to-earth fashion.

1 PHYSICAL DISCOMFORT

The worst source of discomfort during love-making in meno-pausal women is a dry vagina and sore vulva. This, as we saw in Chapter Two, is due to degeneration of the delicate membrane lining these areas as a result of hormonal changes occurring at this time.

The best news in this connection is that sexual activity con-tinuing through and after the menopause actually helps to prevent this degeneration! This was discovered by members of a combined team of gynaecologists and psychiatrists from New Jersey, USA, and reported in JAMA (21), the *Journal of the American Medical Association*, in the spring of 1983. The report was summarized in this country in *Medical News* a month later (22), and aroused much interest and discussion.

The team conducting the trial studied 52 post-menopausal women, with an average age of 57 years. Of these, 25 women were sexually active (having had intercourse a minimum of three times a month over the preceding year), and 23 were inactive (having had intercourse less than ten times in the preceding year). Four women could not be classified.

The active and inactive groups of women were similar in most respects – age, partner's age, years married, age at menarche (onset of periods) and at the commencement of regular menstrua-tion. They were also of comparable educational level, had had similar numbers of vaginal deliveries (i.e. babies delivered nor-mally through the vagina, rather than by Caesarean section), and belonged to the same religion(s).

Only two variable factors were significant in a statistical sense – the inactive women had lower gross incomes, and weighed on average 8.1 kg more than the active women. The premenopausal sexual activities of the two groups had *not* differed.

The Vaginal Atrophy Index (VAI), based on skin elasticity and turgor, the pubic hair, and examination of the labia (vaginal lips), vaginal entrance, vaginal lining membrane and vaginal depth, was evaluated by a gynaecologist for each patient. Overall, significant-ly less degeneration was noted in the sexually active women, and 5 of the 6 VAI factors showed a trend to less degeneration in the women as individuals as well.

Not only was there evidence to prove that frequent sexual intercourse maintains the youthful condition of the genital membranes, there was also every indication that frequent masturbation may be helpful in lieu of actual intercourse.

Another interesting finding was that the women's current frequency of love-making was not significantly related to levels of hormones in the blood, but there were correlations between desire for intercourse (assessed in terms of frequency) and the blood level of male-type sex hormones.

This particular study indicated that female membrane degeneration was *unrelated* to oestrogen levels (contrary to the belief normally held), but that women with little degeneration had raised levels both of androgens (male sex hormones) and of the pituitary hormones LH and FSH (luteinizing hormone and follicle stimulating hormone).

The final deduction from this study was that androgens rather than oestrogens play a role in retarding the ageing of the genital membranes, and that they are critical in the maintenance of interest in sexual intercourse.

You may agree that this study was very interesting for what it was worth. Many doctors still believe that it is the falling level of oestradiol that causes menopausal women to suffer from a dry, sore vagina and itchy vulva. If they are wrong, and it is a low level of male hormone that is responsible, you may wonder how that is going to help since no woman would contemplate taking male sex hormones to buck up her sex drive or keep her membranes youthful.

The relevance of the study here is that – whatever the truth about the hormones – a healthy vaginal membrane is definitely related to frequent love-making. Failing that, it is even correlated with regular masturbation. There is every reason to go on making love as often and as regularly as you conveniently can, and forgetting every taboo you have ever heard about sex not being the done thing after you reach a certain age.

There is no doubt, either, that youthful 'non-degenerating' genital membranes are considerably healthier than ones showing signs of age. The better the condition in which you can keep the lining of your vagina and vulva (see Chapter Two), the less likely you will be to suffer from either the constant itch of pruritus vulvae, or the painful, dry inflammation of kraurosis vulvae.

I must stress here, though, that *any* post-coital bleeding *must* be reported to your doctor as soon as possible. Once your periods have stopped it is emphatically not 'all right' to bleed from the vagina or vulva, either after intercourse or for no apparent reason. Only a full internal examination, which involves a cervical smear, can determine the cause and lead to diagnosis and treatment.

Masturbation, mentioned in the above report, may well be a word you feel should be taboo, and a practice that no self-respecting woman, middle-aged or otherwise, would seriously consider indulging in. If so, at a risk of upsetting you, I am obliged to say, firstly, that masturbation is not the result of a sick mind at work, but the action of a healthy mind and body with normal desires. Secondly, whatever you may believe about its frequency, the majority of women (and men for that matter) *do* masturbate in the privacy of their own bedrooms, and are all the better for doing so.

Of course it is still a socially unacceptable practice in public. We will, it is to be hoped, always continue to explain to small boys and girls that it is better *not* to play and explore 'down there', in front of other people, or at school, or in public conveniences. All the same, we should also continue to make every effort to ensure that they do not feel dirty, unnatural, or ashamed at their perfectly understandable curiosity. They simply have to realize that there are certain places where such investigations are perfectly in order, and others where they are not.

I also recommend masturbation as a normal and excellent means of releasing pent-up emotions, of inducing a warm, comfortable and relaxing sleep (far better for you than sleeping tablets) if practised last thing at night, and of providing yourself with a few minutes of sexual pleasure whenever you fancy it and have the opportunity.

I will be ending this chapter with a few words about sexual technique and foreplay. With respect to immediate relief from a dry vagina and inflamed labia, try applying pure Aloe vera gel morning and night to all the sore parts. This herbal extract is an excellent healer and natural anti-inflammatory agent, and is obtained from a cactus-like plant, the leaves of which are used as a source of Bitter Aloes – sometimes still painted on fingernails as a deterrent against biting. Use the gel as a lubricant, too, before making love, just as you would KY jelly.

2 LACK OF SELF-CONFIDENCE

I have mentioned several different very good reasons why some menopausal women lack self-confidence. They have included putting on weight, the emotional effect of being infertile, a lack of interest in sex and fear of falling personal standards at work or at home, or both.

The worst thing about contributory causes is that most of them aggravate one another and it is very difficult to separate cause and effect. 'Lack of interest in sex', for instance, may be the reason for putting on weight (i.e. at a subconscious level 'If I put on weight I won't be attractive to him, so he'll cease to bother me.' Or the connection might be more direct, i.e. lack of sexual desire leads to no love-making, and therefore a whole host of emotional needs go unfulfilled. Result? Eating sugary snacks and junk food for comfort).

To illustrate the complexity of the problem, you can just as legitimately invert the issue. A menopausal woman finds her weight going up and, instead of eating wholefood and exercising, she does what so many obesity victims do, and eats to comfort herself – realizing full well the inevitable result. Loathing the look of herself, she 'loses interest in sex', because secretly she cannot bring herself to let her husband see her undressed in her present state.

Compound this situation – or a hundred variations on this

theme – with frequent hot flushes, fatigue from sleepless nights, intense irritability and constant indigestion (from all the secret Mars bar stuffing) and it is easy to see why menopausal difficulties can appear an almost inextricable mixture of physical and mental problems.

One has to pick up a thread somewhere, though, to reach the centre of the maze, and an invariably safe one to take hold of, when looking for reasons for a lack of self-confidence, is appearance. Every woman knows the truth of the magazine cliché 'to feel good you have to look good' – at least in your own eyes – and having seen some of the misery ageing skin, extra pounds of fat and dull hair can cause, I would put attention to appearance close to the top of my list of priorities.

A wholefood diet, with the supplements I have recommended, and regular exercise will improve the circulation, and thereby the complexion; reduce excess weight and keep it steady; cause eyes to sparkle, hair to become lustrous, and fingernails to stop splitting. If you cannot wait for all this magic effect to take place, here are some extra supplements to help you with specific problems.

(i) To lose weight

The amino acids arginine and ornithine stimulate the pituitary gland to produce growth hormone (GH). Usually its secretion of this hormone falls off sharply at the end of the growing years. The effect of GH secretion in the fully formed adult is to help him or her regain a slim, firm and lean physique.

Other factors stimulating the pituitary gland in this way are sleep, exercise and fasting (the latter should only be undertaken at the advice and under the supervision of a health professional).

The best time to take the two amino acids is at bedtime, on an empty stomach, with water or fruit juice. Recommended doses differ somewhat according to the research findings consulted, but some that are used are: arginine 1200 mg, ornithine 900 mg. Sometimes the amino acid lysine is recommended too (1200 mg dose).

These amino acid supplements are available to the public but it is considered to be more satisfactory to consult a nutritionist who will supervise your amino acid dietary supplementation personally.

(ii) For falling hair
The stress B complex in your daily supplement programme will help this problem — your mineral supplements of calcium and magnesium should be at least 1000 mg and 500 mg respectively. In addition, choline and inositol intake should be 1000 mg each. Finally, a daily jojoba oil scalp massage and shampoo.

(iii) Skin wrinkles
PABA (see Chapter Six) is a B vitamin, and is said both to help restore natural colour to the hair and to delay the formation of skin wrinkles. Good B-complex supplements contain PABA in doses of 30 to 100 mg. The recommended dose for this effect is up to 100 mg three times daily.

(iv) Splitting fingernails
If you have not included Efamol in your daily regimen and want to cure splitting, flaking fingernails, add three capsules twice a day.

When lack of self-confidence stems from poor memory and concentration in addition to a dowdy appearance, it can help to supplement the diet with lecithin; a convenient form is the granules available in tins as Lecigran in health food shops — take two tablespoonfuls a day. This supplies a very useful supplement in this context — phosphatidyl choline — as well as phosphatidyl inositol.

3 REPRESSED AGGRESSION AND FEAR
Considering the self-doubts and the physical discomfort that it is possible to experience during the menopause if you eat the wrong diet, never exercise, encounter lots of stress factors every day and suffer from a sore vagina, it is hardly surprising menopausal women get irritable. Irritability also seems to be a symptom in its

own right at this time, rather as tension is a typical feature of the premenstrual syndrome.

There is no doubt, though, that hidden anger and fear play a large part in causing outbreaks of aggression which can, incidentally, come as much as a surprise to the woman herself as to her friends and colleagues on the receiving end. Emotions – for a variety of reasons – are more unstable then, and it takes very little to spark off an outburst you regret later.

The soundest advice I can give to any menopausal woman feeling waves of boundless anger rise up inside is to talk about your feelings! The best person to discuss this with is the man you live with. If you are snappy and bad-tempered it would put his mind at rest for you to admit that some of it is your fault. And if you have been harbouring resentment and irritation for years about petty little habits he has, now is the time to bring them out into the open.

He may change, or he may not! The important thing is that *you* are changing things for yourself, by bringing to the surface resentment and anger that, left there for much longer, could undermine all your other efforts to start life afresh. Once you have voiced small problems, you will be able to see them for what they are. Left alone for years to fester, small worries and resentments permit little time for inner tranquillity and magnify the effects of other, unavoidable stress factors out of all proportion.

If you feel you have emotional or psychological problems with which you cannot cope, and which yoga, autogenics or self-hypnosis fail to resolve, then I suggest you obtain some outside help. I do recommend that you go privately to see a therapist, if you can possibly manage to do so. Your doctor could refer you to the psychiatric department of your local hospital – but the demands upon psychiatrists' time are such that they are permitted very little time indeed per patient. Certainly not long enough – most of them would freely admit – really to sort out complex emotional and psychological problems, and give their patients adequate psychotherapy on a regular basis. Frequently, all that time allows is fifteen to twenty minutes of discussion, and just when you are beginning to relax and explain yourself properly, it's the end of the appointment and you find yourself being offered a prescription for either tranquillizers or an anti-depressant. This is far from ideal – and the chances are slim that you will see the original doctor at the next appointment, or even ever again.

My own recommendation is that you seek out a hypnotherapist. Stress reactions and anxiety, coupled with a chronic inability to relax, lie at the heart of very many psychological disturbances, phobias and anxieties that arise in women in their forties and fifties. Hypnotherapists are of course especially well-qualified to help you learn the art of relaxation – and many patients find that an hour a week spent simply in talking to a sympathetic listener is highly therapeutic in itself.

Hypnotherapists are qualified to deal with depression and anxiety, phobic fears, unwanted habits such as drinking problems, smoking and nail-biting, compulsive activities such as having to repeat an action several times over to release worry, and psychosomatic illnesses in which you experience a number of very real symptoms for which no doctor can find a cause.

Love Making

Now you are aware of the advantages of revamping your own attitude to life, and that means your lifestyle as well, do make an effort to improve your love life if you feel that it is less than ideal. You may well have spent the past six months (or years) pleading headaches just before bedtime – and your husband may well have got the message to leave you alone – but it is just possible that neither of you is exactly delighted with the present state of affairs.

If you haven't talked about the subject for a very long time (but you would secretly like to do so), open the discussion as casually as you can, when you are both alone together. I have already talked about sex therapy for couples with a definable sexual problem, so the kind of situation I am picturing here is that of sexual shyness and 'just having got out of the habit'.

A relaxed setting is essential. I am not suggesting that you shock the poor man by wafting downstairs wearing nothing but Opium next time you get him to yourself. But there is everything to be said for making *some* effort, such as cooking him his favourite meal, buying a bottle of wine, and switching the TV off.

It is easier under these conditions to talk about good times you've had together, fun you have shared, holidays you have been on, and, yes, pleasures in bed you have both enjoyed. If all this sounds too heavy – *you* are the expert, and you know your man. Lead up to the subject any way you like and anywhere. But if you want to get down to business on the subject of love-making, pick the right moment!

If it's present technique that is worrying you, do say so! Most men take suggestions of change as a personal criticism of themselves – so gently point out that it is nothing of the kind. Flatter him where you can do so sincerely – and ask him to be slower, more gentle, spend longer in foreplay, play with you in the shower first – feel free to ask him anything you like!

The most important message about the menopause is that it is a new beginning – and in no way more so than in sexual matters. If you are having problems getting an orgasm, stop faking them (gradually) and say you need his help. Awaken his sense of chivalry (apparently all men have at least a vestige of this; it is inherited as part of the evolutionary process) and once you can make him feel needed, the missing warmth and familiarity will soon rekindle into passion and pleasure.

Chapter Eight

Throwing out unwanted habits

Most of us have a habit or two we would be pleased to be rid of. Since the menopause is a time for changes in the most positive sense, it would be a great pity if you altered your lifestyle in the ways I have recommended, yet continued, for instance, to smoke, to drink too much alcohol, or to rely on drugs you would be better off without.

Smoking

If you are a smoker, the chances are that you have already tried to break your addiction to cigarettes. Some smokers do, of course, persist in smoking no matter what, protesting that cigarettes are one of their few pleasures, and that they are sure that *they* will not develop lung cancer as a result.

This opinion is often based on having had a relative or friend who has smoked heavily until the age of ninety without apparently suffering any ill effects. Unfortunately, it is false reasoning to assume that the same good luck will apply to oneself. Cancer has no respect for age, sex or illusions of safety -- and can just as easily develop after twenty or thirty symptom-free years of smoking, as it can within the first few.

In addition, lung cancer is only one of the possible ill effects associated with the repeated inhalation of nicotine, coal tar and related poisons. Carcinoma of the large bowel, the mouth and tongue, and possibly the breast and cervix are all now believed to be linked with the habit. Other possibly fatal disorders directly related to it include heart disease, especially coronary thrombosis (heart attack); arterial disease and thrombosis; and strokes. Varicose veins, varicose eczema and varicose ulcers are definitely made worse by smoking, as are some peptic ulcers and hiatus hernias, recurrent asthma attacks, hay fever, sinusitis and chronic catarrh.

There is another especially good reason to quit smoking when you reach the menopause if you have not already done so. The fact that women during their reproductive years suffer far fewer heart attacks and far less arterial disease than men has been attributed to the oestrogen they secrete. Since the level of ovarian oestrogen declines markedly at the menopause, this protective effect does not exist for women from the time of the menopause onwards. If you add to this incentive to stop the fact that the incidence of lung cancer among women is rising yearly, you will find every encouragement to make the effort required.

The various products available on the market to help you quit cigarettes include cassette tapes available by mail order and often at chemist shops; herbal remedies, advertised in health magazines and also available from chemists; and nicotine chewing gum (Nicorette) available from your doctor on prescription.

Alternative therapies likely to help you stop smoking include hypnotherapy; acupuncture; and an aversion technique available at certain health farms and on a private basis. Self-help techniques include yoga and meditation; and autohypnosis. Autogenics is sometimes very useful – see Chapter Five. You can direct your attention to tingles in your throat and chest or any other withdrawal symptoms you get, learning to 'switch them off' whenever they are about to bother you. Biofeedback is also a likely aid in this respect.

Eating Too Much

I believe that people in developed countries are divided into two groups with respect to their eating habits. There are those to whom food matters very much indeed, and whose thoughts fly instantly to fish and chips or a whole box of *marrons glacés* the moment life becomes stressful. And there are the others who undoubtedly suffer as much from the effects of stress as the first group, but who turn to different sources of comfort when the world mistreats them.

Not surprisingly, men and women belonging to the first group tend to be overweight. Those in the second rarely are, at least not as a result of over-eating. They may refuse to exercise, drink like fishes, and end up gigantic in size. But at least they do not have to contend with the constant 'Tussle of the Biscuit Tin', in which every waking moment for days on end is plagued by unquench-able yearnings for sugary, starchy junk food snacks.

If you belong to the first group – and I must admit I do – you should be encouraged by the news that the wholefood diet and exercise regimen I suggest in this book can overcome the problem for you if you let them. And I do not simply mean that if you eat a lot of salad and pulses and wholewheat spaghetti, you won't have room for unhealthy, calorie-ridden extras. As every food addict knows, 'room' has little to do with the issue.

What actually happens is that the craving for non-wholefood products gradually vanishes. If you doubt the truth of this, I can tell you that I was sceptical when I read about this effect in *Raw Energy* (23). Leslie and Susannah Kenton claim that eating a high raw diet gradually curbs addictive cravings for fattening food items, but it was not until I altered my own way of eating that I discovered the truth for myself.

I had been eating a wholefood diet, between 60 and 70% of which consisted of raw vegetables, fruit, grains and seeds, when I suddenly realized that I had not eaten a Mars bar for at least a fortnight. Neither had I raided the biscuit tin, or had a midnight snack of buttered toast and marmalade. I have had the occasional bar of chocolate since then, but to be perfectly honest, I have not really enjoyed it.

Another factor that helps to curb the desire to binge is exercise. Daily exercise over and above a certain minimum amount stimulates the appetite-regulating centre in the brain (the 'appestat'), with which mechanism many overweight sedentary people lose contact in their late twenties. The re-awakening of this physiological reflex means that 'stop!' signals are once more transmitted to our conscious minds when we have taken in enough calories to cope with our energy output. We no longer feel like stuffing ourselves, and cravings become a thing of the past.

I have already given details of dietary supplements that aid weight loss. If you would like a further dietary supplement that curbs the appetite naturally, in the place of appetite suppressant drugs, then I recommend that you try the amino acid phenylalanine. This suppresses appetite by releasing a chemical substance known as CCK (cholecystokinin), believed to induce a sensation of satiety, possibly by interacting with the central nervous system feeding centres. The dose of phenylalanine is between 100 and 500 mg per day, either in divided doses prior to meals, or on an empty stomach before retiring. Its side effects are bonuses and include improved mental alertness, better memory, increased interest in sex and after 24 to 48 hours, an anti-depressant effect. It is interesting to compare the side effects of this amino acid with those of standard appetite suppressant drugs mentioned later on in this chapter.

For serious overeating problems, which resist all attempts to overcome them through exercise, wholefood diet and relaxation techniques, I would recommend that you try group therapy (Weight Watchers, Successful Slimming clubs). If even these don't help you gain control of your eating urges, then I suggest you have some private psychotherapy treatment if you can afford it — preferably hypnotherapy because of its emphasis upon learning to relax.

Drinking Too Much

Many of my above remarks about over-eating apply equally to over-drinking. There are certain important differences, however, that should be mentioned, the first being the greater subtlety with which alcohol becomes a problem in the first place. However serious a threat obesity poses to health, fatness is still a topic about which many jokes are made, and over-eating a habit to which many plump people readily admit.

Drinking too much, by contrast, still has a stigma attached to it. Women, in particular, are likely to be slow in admitting, even to themselves, that they have any kind of a problem with alcohol. Imperceptibly the desire for a drink can develop into the need for one – and the next temptation to present itself is often the buying and hiding of a secret supply of wine or spirits. The usual motivation is the avoidance of the questions, accusations and rows that often develop when one partner begins to drink more heavily than usual. It can also be a sign of growing dependence, and one that demands your attention and concern.

There is not room here to enter fully into alcohol dependence. The best advice I can give is for you to discuss any problem you may think you have in this direction either with your partner, a reliable friend, your parents or doctor. Try cutting out alcohol altogether, say for three days a week, and then confining it to weekends.

If this does not work, psychotherapy or group therapy (Alcoholics Anonymous) are very helpful indeed and I cannot recommend them, especially the latter, too highly. While you are working out your problem, do keep taking the dietary supplements recommended in Chapter Six. Remember in particular to include Efamol, three 500 mg capsules three times a day. As well as helping to avoid hangovers, Efamol affords the liver valuable protection against the effects of excess alcohol.

Drug Dependence

This section is not as inappropriate as it sounds. No one is suggesting for a moment that many – or perhaps any – menopausal women spend their free afternoons mainlining heroin, or sniffing cocaine. Nevertheless, there is a tremendous amount of dependence throughout all age groups upon the so-called harmless drugs such as tranquillizers and sleeping tablets. And it is not hard to see how the menopause – if mishandled – can increase this dependence in a number of directions.

What I intend to do here is to look at the several groups of drugs which are commonly over-prescribed, and suggest, where I can, possible ways of cutting down your intake, or doing without them altogether.

TRANQUILLIZERS
Common tranquillizers include diazepam (the notorious Valium); chlordiazepoxide (Librium); lorazepam (Ativan); meprobamate (Equanil). Like the vast majority of drugs, they all have their uses and their good points, and often get an undeservedly bad press – chiefly because the passion for 'alternatives' tends to condemn as harmful toxins any medicines that do not actually grow wild.

The main problem with tranquillizers is that they are frequently prescribed for the wrong reasons. Valium and Librium can be very useful, say, following severe emotional shock, such as bereavement – given in small doses, and for a week or ten days only. What happens, though, is that the doctor prescribes, say, 5 mg tablets where the 2 mg strength would be adequate, supplies enough for a month, and repeats the prescription on request – often without actually seeing the patient.

Much of the underlying problem is the little time doctors have available for each patient. The solution is to make known the alternatives that are available and that actually *work*, so that doctors can advise their patients to turn to natural remedies as and when these are appropriate.

You know you are dependent upon a tranquillizer when you

feel ill enough on stopping the tablets to start taking them again. Ativan, Librium and Valium are all capable of causing dependence, and this can arise in susceptible people within a few weeks on a course of tablets – it is not necessary to take them for months or years to find that you cannot do without them.

I hope I have said enough in this book so far to convince you of the physically and mentally stabilizing effects of whole, natural foods with a high component of raw ingredients, of regular aerobic exercise (*excellent* for stress and tension), and of relaxation techniques such as yoga and autohypnosis.

Try psychotherapy or hypnotherapy, rather than take tranquillizers. If you do find yourself on a course of them, take them for as short a time as possible. If you are trying to get off them, check with your doctor and try the natural sedative effect of a herbal remedy such as Quiet Life tablets, available from health food shops. Alternatively, seek out a homoeopathic remedy, either (preferably) by visiting a homoeopathic practitioner, or by buying a remedy for anxiety.

Ask your health food shop manager about the different types. Two that are sometimes prescribed for anxiety and panic attacks are Aconite, and Arsen. Alb. (Arsenicum Album). The dose is two tablets for an adult, every two hours in acute conditions, for six doses; then three times a day between meals for three days. In cases of chronic anxiety, take two tablets three times a day until relief is obtained. Watch your response to the tablets and when you notice some relief, increase the intervals between the doses, continuing for two days more only. Then stop, repeating only if the original symptoms recur.

ANTI-DEPRESSANTS

Most of my remarks about tranquillizers apply equally to anti-depressant tablets. They can be useful for a short time, but it is essential that, instead of coming to rely on them, you (possibly with psychotherapeutic help) discover the reason for your depression and do something constructive about it.

Popular anti-depressants (from the doctor's point of view)

include the tricyclic anti-depressants (e.g. nortriptyline – Allegron; clomipramine – Anafranil; imipramine – Tofranil); and the MAOIs, or monoamine oxidase inhibitors – tranylcypromine (Parnate), phenelzine (Nardil), and isocarboxazid (Marplan). You know if you are taking an MAOI, even if you cannot read the name of the drug on the bottle, because you will have been told to avoid certain dietary items, such as broad bean pods, red wine, blue cheese and other yeast or fungus containing foods, and pickled herring (this is not a complete list).

There is a supplement that can help tide you over the worst patches of depression, without your having to take a drug; it doesn't work for every single person who takes it, but it helps a good many – so much so that it is also made now by pharmaceutical firms under the name of Optimax and Pacitron. The natural supplement is the amino acid tryptophan, and you are better off buying this in an additive-free form from your health food shop as this will be 100% natural. A daily intake of three grams of this amino acid, together with one gram of nicotinamide (a form of vitamin B3), was found in one trial to have better effects upon depressed patients than ECT (electroconvulsive therapy), administered twice weekly. Other trials have shown variable results, but some of these variations are thought to have been due to too small numbers of depressed patients taking part in the trials, and to the relative numbers of different types of depressed people included in the trials, whose reactions to tryptophan might vary.

Do not take tryptophan with a protein meal, but do try to take it together with a small carbohydrate meal or snack. A glass of freshly squeezed carrot juice or a wholemeal biscuit and glass of orange juice would be ideal. Add to this your daily pyridoxine supplement (vitamin B6) as this helps your body to make maximum use of tryptophan. Do *not* take it if you are pregnant, or on monoamine oxidase inhibitors (see above).

SLEEPING TABLETS
You can stop taking these as well if you wish to do so – even if you

have had two Mogadon (nitrazepam), Euhypnos (temazepam) or Noctec (chloral hydrate) capsules every night for the last ten years. Wean yourself off them gradually (this remark applies to all drugs you wish to stop taking) and let your GP know what you are doing. Start by halving the dose, and if this is impossible because they are in capsule form and you only take one anyway, take a capsule on alternate nights and see how you fare.

At the same time, save up your relaxation exercises to do just before you go to bed. If you use autohypnosis the chances are that you will go off into pleasant, natural sleep anyway, instead of 'coming back up' from your trance. Sip a warm drink in bed, or try freshly squeezed vegetable juice – carrot and lettuce mixed is a natural sedative.

There are many herbal remedies that will help you to sleep naturally. If you are taking tryptophan for depression, this will help you to sleep soundly and to fall asleep more quickly than you usually do. Take it half an hour before bed, at least an hour after eating protein food. The herbalist Maurice Messegué recommends (24) his special 'tea of happiness' as an inducer of sound sleep (and also as a remedy for anxiety). It consists of adding two pinches of each of the following herbs (available if you live in a town from your health food shop) to a litre (1¾ pints) of water – vervain, mint, lime flowers and camomile. One cup nightly. If you do not like the taste of this, try a cup of plain camomile tea just before retiring.

APPETITE SUPPRESSANTS

Most people know of the dangers involved in taking drugs of this type. Fibre-based products that fill you up artificially are safe enough, but irrelevant to you if you eat a wholefood diet that includes a high proportion of raw foods.

The dangers are associated with the chemical appetite suppressants, such as diethylpropion (Tenuate Dospan, Apisate) which, like the drug amphetamine which gave rise to them, are highly addictive and cause great mental alertness as well as a diminished appetite. Patients in fact report a variety of effects – some feel 'floaty' and unreal, others get a great 'lift' and feel high, and others eat as usual and experience nothing whatever.

Enough people do get high on them, though, for them to have been soundly abused in the past, and they are now on the limited list which means that they are harder for your GP to prescribe.

Phenylalanine (see above) is safe and does increase mental alertness, without producing a dramatic 'high' or causing any type of addiction.

OTHER DRUGS

A final few words about drugs you don't normally think of as being over-prescribed. Tablets for high blood pressure account for a large fraction of the total number of prescriptions written every week of the year. Typically, blood pressure rises in association with increased body weight in men and women in their forties and fifties onwards. Do not just stop taking blood pressure medication – especially if you tend to have moderately severe blood pressure problems. But let your GP know that you would be keen to have the dose reduced and maybe even stop taking them altogether, providing you can manage to keep your blood pressure down unaided by his medications.

The way to do this is to reduce your body weight to normal, along the lines I have already suggested. It is also helpful to use a relaxation technique daily, and to direct part of the technique towards the lowering of blood pressure. This is where autogenics or autohypnosis, backed up by weekly or twice weekly yoga sessions, could help. Biofeedback would also be especially relevant here.

Lastly, laxatives, a highly abused form of drug, especially when bought over the counter! Laxatives are fine for very occasional use – but using them every day, or even very often, is very bad for your large bowel (colon). The more it is 'helped' to work, the more reliant it becomes on the aid of laxatives, and the greater your need for laxatives becomes.

When you change to a high raw, wholefood diet, there should be absolutely no need for laxatives – and no need for adding bran to everything as you will be taking in ample raw fibre to stimulate your bowel naturally. Stop taking whatever you are used to taking in this line and let your bowel resume its normal function – which it will ultimately do, given the opportunity.

Chapter Nine

Alternative treatments can help

It is highly likely that the lifestyle changes so far suggested in this book will put an end to your menopausal symptoms and, I hope, make you feel happier, more confident and about ten years younger! Should you continue, despite this, to suffer from hot flushes, headaches, periodic depression or any of the other minor disorders capable of plaguing the menopausal years, then I suggest you seek further help along the following lines.

First and foremost, see your doctor if you have the least doubt about the significance of a persistent symptom. Only you can judge whether this is necessary, but do remember that your GP is the best person to put your mind at rest with respect to diagnosis. This is not to deny for a moment the probable validity of alternative diagnostic techniques such as iridology or electrocrystal diagnosis; but even practitioners of these methods generally prefer to complement orthodox diagnosis rather than to try to replace it altogether.

I cannot emphasize too strongly the necessity of going for a check up if you notice a breast lump or post-coital (i.e. post-intercourse) bleeding; if you start to bleed again from the vagina for any other reason, once your periods are over; or if you suffer from, say, recurrent severe headaches, deep depression or alcohol/ cigarette addiction.

When a diagnosis has been reached, and your mind set at rest, you can then consult an alternative practitioner to see what additional help is available. If all your GP is able to offer you is repeat prescriptions for tablets, then you may well decide to try alternative therapy in conjunction with your medication, with a view to tailing off the orthodox treatment as soon as possible.

Types of alternative therapy you might like to try, should the need arise, include naturopathy, acupuncture, homoeopathy and reflexology. Hypnotherapy has already been discussed, and several herbal remedies mentioned.

1 Naturopathy

You could really say that the whole approach of this book is naturopathic. Naturopathy is based on the principle that the body can heal itself of disorders, given the right conditions. The naturopathic doctor sees illness as resulting from disharmony within, brought about by unnatural and injurious lifestyle habits adversely affecting the homoeostatic mechanism.

Rectify bad habits, he maintains, and the body's natural powers of healing will be able to function normally, restoring inner balance and complete health.

The first of his patient's 'habits' the naturopath attends to is generally diet. Fasting, and the excretion from the system of accumulated toxins, play important roles in much naturopathic practice, but the fasting is carefully monitored by the practitioner and is generally modified by permitting the consumption of freshly squeezed fruit and vegetable juice.

Fasting, or semi-fasting, is often combined with 'skin brushing', which accelerates the loss of toxic waste through the skin. For this you will be shown how to use a long-handled, natural bristle brush such as the type you use in the bath for scrubbing your back. To carry out this technique, you brush every area of your skin, with the exception of your face, moderately firmly, working from the soles of your feet upwards.

When you get to your abdominal area, gently sweep the skin surface with the brush, using a clockwise motion (i.e. the direction of the large bowel, or colon, as it runs up the right side of the abdomen, along the top below the ribs and down the left hand side to the rectum). When you have finished your skin brush, take a warm shower followed by a few seconds of cold shower.

The type of diet a naturopathic doctor will suggest will undoubtedly be a wholefood one, with a high raw food content, modified in whatever way(s) he or she sees fit to suit you as an individual. He will decide upon these in the course of taking a full case history, much importance being attached to the consultation, as indeed it is by the practitioners of most alternative forms of medicine.

Any possible allergies to food or environmental factors may become apparent during the case history, and if the practitioner seeks further information on the subject of allergic reactions, he may suggest your referral to a clinical ecologist or to a kinesiologist. (Both of these types of professional specialize in the detection of allergy.)

Lifestyle changes, particularly with respect to regular exercise, relaxation techniques and the cessation of injurious habits such as smoking and excessive drinking, would be suggested to you. Special attention would be paid to stress factors to which you are subject, and advice given about the best way to cope with these.

Where the naturopathic doctor saw fit, he might co-operate with a herbalist, a homoeopath, an osteopath or an acupuncturist to provide additional relief from symptoms.

Some naturopaths favour dietary supplements, others do not. Those who do would be sure to recommend that you take natural forms of the necessary vitamins, minerals and other compounds to ensure that you avoid absorbing artificial fillers, dyes, flavourings and other synthetics.

2 Acupuncture

Like naturopathic philosophy, acupuncture is based on the principle of the body's innate ability to heal itself, if it is provided with the correct stimuli. Practitioners see health as dependent upon the

harmonious integration of two opp
forces, Yin and Yang.

Unlike blood pressure, temperatu
two forces are not directly measur
bear more resemblance to the elen
natural universe – such as water,
darkness (Yin qualities), and fire, su
qualities).

Although certain body organs are more 'Yin
instance, the womb, the vagina), and others more 'Yan
penis), overall balance throughout the body of the two factors is
what determines health or disease. The various representative
organs and body areas of Yin and Yang are in a continual state of
flux, the balance between the two being in a state of dynamic
equilibrium.

Obviously, the balance constantly fluctuates a little in one
direction and then a little in the other. If the sum total of
'Yang-ness', however, finally overcomes the sum total of 'Yin-
ness', disharmony is established and the health becomes dis-
ordered.

This way of looking at anatomy, physiology and biochemistry
may seem very odd to us, but if you think of Yin and Yang
harmony as representing what we refer to as homoeostasis, the
concept becomes far easier to accept. Homoeostasis is the Western idea of physiological and biochemical balance, and its attain-
ment and maintenance in terms of body temperature, blood
acidity or alkalinity, blood glucose levels and hormone output,
constitute collectively a simple definition of health.

The practical application of Yin and Yang philosophy determines precisely how the two forces are out of harmony, and what
disorder has resulted from the imbalance. The forces are then
rebalanced by the application of the right stimuli (acupuncture
needling techniques) and a cure is effected.

Even this brief and simplistic account of acupuncture would be
incomplete without mention of the meridians or energy channels
that are fundamental to the art. These are a system of pathways

the body that distribute Qi or natural energy to the
gans. Disturbance or cessation of an energy pathway
e energy flow inside it occurs when Yin and Yang are out
nce, so that a disorder arises.

upuncture points are focal points along the meridians, repre-
ting the position of maximum influence upon the flow of Qi
ithin. It is at a selection of these points that acupuncture needles
are applied, with the object of repairing the damaged meridian
and restoring the normal flow of energy.

Regarding what you may expect acupuncture to do for you, the
following symptoms and disorders are likely to respond. Aches
and pains may be due to muscular tension, and may disappear as
soon as you start to take more exercise and to learn to relax
properly.

On the other hand, lack of beneficial exercise, excessive weight
and poor posture may have contributed to definable muscular
strain, early osteoarthritis, fibrositis and other forms of muscular
rheumatism. Acupuncture may be useful in all of these, most work
having been done in the field of pain relief for osteoarthritis, in
which the pain relief lasts from between six months to two years
(25).

Headaches, anxiety, depression, digestive problems such as
peptic ulceration and gall stones (these typically appear in women
in their forties and fifties), palpitations, raised blood pressure,
obesity, smoking and drug addiction are also likely to respond to
acupuncture therapy. Finally, hot flushes, night sweats, vaginal
soreness and irritation, and general fatigue (26) have also been
reported as responsive to this therapy.

3 Homoeopathy

This medical discipline, in contrast to acupuncture, arose as a
recognized and discrete system of medicine in eighteenth-century
Germany, and should therefore be more comprehensible to the
Western mind than concepts involving Qi energy, Yin and Yang,

and meridian pathways. Despite this, relatively few people claim to understand precisely how it works.

The principles of homoeopathy illustrate another variation on the theme of health as reflecting inner harmony. The symptoms produced by a certain disease indicate not the passive protestations of a besieged organism, but active resistance on behalf of the individual's homoeostatic mechanism which is striving to overcome the disease process and re-establish harmony.

Far from attempting to dampen these efforts, therefore, homoeopathy seeks to encourage them. Thankfully for the patient, this does not consist of actually intensifying the symptoms from which he is suffering, although this can happen to a slight extent at the commencement of treatment. Homoeopathic remedies are chosen for the similarity of the symptoms that they *would* produce, if given to a healthy person, to those of which the patient is presently complaining.

Thus, an illness whose symptoms started suddenly and featured a high temperature and flushed face, throbbing earache, boils or headache and a fast pulse, would very likely be treated with Atropa belladonna. The reason is that this compound, derived from the Deadly Nightshade, produces very similar symptoms (flushed face, pounding pulse, illness of sudden onset) in a healthy individual who accidentally becomes poisoned with the berries of this plant. The underlying principle of this reasoning is a very old one, and is expressed in Latin as: 'Similia similibus curentur', which means: 'Let likes be treated by likes.'

What can be rather more difficult to understand is the concept of potentization. Samuel Hahnemann, the founder of modern homoeopathic medicine, gave the remedies he used in producing similar symptoms in smaller quantities than were usual for medication doses at that time. He increased a given dose just to the point at which toxic symptoms started to appear, and then he decreased it until they disappeared again.

He started to favour smaller and smaller doses in a desire to do away entirely with toxic side effects, and his dilution of remedies grew naturally from this wish. Eventually, he achieved extremely small doses by a process he called 'potentization', having found in many cases, that the smaller the dose, the greater the beneficial effect.

Of great importance to the homoeopathic method is the sum total of the symptoms displayed by a particular patient. Very detailed questions are asked about all the patient is feeling, both in terms of the actual physical symptoms and in terms of how the disorder is affecting him or her emotionally and psychologically. The appropriate remedy is only chosen after all possible consideration has been given to the complete range of symptoms, and this frequently results in two people suffering from the same complaint (from the orthodox point of view) being treated with different remedies.

Here are two examples of how remedies are chosen according to patient type as well as according to the symptoms they display. Taken from the section of a homoeopathic handbook dealing with the treatment of menopausal symptoms, Pulsatilla is recommended for menopausal women 'who are fair and blue-eyed'. For menopausal women who are dark-haired, on the other hand, Sepia is suggested.

Since homoeopathy is a complete system of medicine, it is reasonable to visit a homoeopathic practitioner for any of the menopausal symptoms discussed in this book – always with the proviso that potentially serious disorders that could mean cancer are discussed with your doctor first. As you will be aware by now, these include the recommencement of uterine or vaginal bleeding, and the discovery of lumps anywhere in or on your body. Any homoeopathic doctor would be in full agreement with this advice.

4 Reflexology

Another name for reflexology is 'compression massage'. It consists of compression or finger massage applied to the feet, and like acupuncture its practice was founded several thousand years BC.

Its practice in the West, however, is of far shorter duration. Dr W. Fitzgerald's discovery in the 1920s that the body is divided into 'zones' of energy led to the development of pressure techniques applied to these areas for both preventive and curative purposes (27). This developed into the modern art and science of reflexology, which has much in common with the methods utilized in ancient China.

Reflexologists recognize a 'life force' which flows along ten conduits in the body that begin in the toes and end elsewhere at the body's upper extremities. These channels may be loosely compared with the meridians of acupuncture, and the life force itself with Qi energy. Again, disorders of the body are attributed to blockage and disruption of the energy flow, the object of the massage being the restoration of the normal and unimpeded energy stream.

Every energy conduit in reflexology is related to a body zone, and to the organs within that zone. An area on the inner aspect of each heel, for example, relates to the uterus (or to the prostate gland in a man); while a spot in a similar position on the outer aspect of the heel, relates to the ovary (or testicle).

By examining the feet with the tips of the fingers, the therapist can elicit 'trouble areas' within the body, i.e. he can determine which energy conduits are blocked. The disorder is rectified by releasing the blocked energy by means of massage of the appropriate area of the foot. Pressure on the appropriate conduit terminals in the feet acts as a stimulus resulting in a reflex that affects the appropriate organ.

A summary of the possible effects of this stimulation includes: 'removing waste deposits, congestion and blockages in the energy pathways, improving blood circulation and gland function, and relaxing the whole system, including the mind' (28).

To the examining fingers of the practitioner, the areas of energy blockage feel like tiny, hard crystals below the skin. Once located, they are broken up by the application of digital pressure. The remaining fragments of waste matter are then absorbed into the tissue fluid and blood stream, and excreted through the body's normal excretory mechanisms such as the urine and the sweat.

As pleasant as foot massage can be under other circumstances (many people – apart from exceptionally ticklish individuals – find having their feet stroked highly erotic), deep pressure applied by a reflexologist can be extremely painful. This pain, however, is said to have the 'unbearable but pleasant' quality of the type resulting from having an inflamed muscle massaged. Patients grimace at the discomfort but say that they can 'feel it doing them good'.

Like all other alternative practitioners, reflexologists see stress reactions and inner tension as a common cause of energy blockage. One well-known reflexology expert in the USA – Eunice D. Ingham – believed that one can 'choke off a portion of the normal blood supply to various parts of the body by refusing to stop needless worry' (29). She felt that both worry and anger can bring about the formation of the channel blocking crystals.

There are few disorders that reflexologists feel cannot be assisted by this speciality. It is particularly recommended for overcoming chronic tension and inducing a deep inner tranquillity. Poor sleeping habits respond favourably, and common menopausal problems listed in the index of a well-known book written by two reflexologists: *Reflexology. Techniques of Foot Massage for Health and Fitness* include hot flushes, emotional stress, fatigue, headaches and being overweight (28).

Chapter Ten

A fulfilling future

The menopause is an excellent time to start life afresh. If I seem to be repeating that message over and over again, it is because it is the most important piece of information that this book can convey. There is a saying that 'life begins at forty'. So much the better if you make the necessary improvements then. But if you take the menopause as the marking point of a new, healthy and satisfying lifestyle, then you can make the event something to look forward to, rather than to dread.

With respect to the actual changes I suggest, it is important that you do not attempt to make them all at once. If you do feel the need to alter several aspects of your life simultaneously, at least make sure that you approach your objectives gradually, and refuse to be put off by minor failures.

You may think this advice is erring on the side of caution, because all I have basically advised you to do is to eat a supplemented wholefood diet, take regular exercise, adopt a relaxation technique and think about improving your sex life. The sum total of this does not sound momentous, but old habits are renowned for their staying power, and there is nothing more depressing than seeing all your recent good intentions go sailing down the drain 'yet again'.

Wholefood Diet

Take a wholefood diet, for instance. Few people, if any, would stick to this way of eating if they did not enjoy it – even nutritional experts who are more aware than most of us of the reasons for avoiding junk food.

'Whole' ingredients provide delicious, satisfying meals, that are more flavourful than any of the attractively wrapped processed convenience foods you can buy. They also provide the basis for excellent and sophisticated dinner party menus, and are especially appreciated by cooks who rely upon simple ingredients of superlative quality and freshness. You have only to read Sarah Brown's books (30) to be convinced of that.

If you try to switch overnight, though, from white, sliced bread to homemade wholemeal, from butter to margarine, and from your Sunday roast to grilled herrings (for their EPA content) your family will make for the nearest pub, and even you will find the changes too much of a contrast!

Buy wrapped Hovis, for example, before starting to make your own 100% wholemeal loaves. Use Krona margarine, or Blue Band, which really do taste quite like butter, for a month or so before buying one of the brands with a high polyunsaturate content (Vitaquell).

Also, start looking at the recipes in the two leading health magazines (*Here's Health* and *New Health*). Their cookery writers know all about the problems of feeding large families wholefood diets that please them, and also about the need to produce attractive meals and snacks speedily and cheaply. A feature that appeared quite recently in one of these magazines even gave recipes for nutritionally satisfactory fish and chips! And recipes abound for delicious cakes, puddings, flans, hors d'oeuvres and main courses. So there is no need to make a change to wholefood eating a life of self-denial.

Supplements

I suggest that you make small changes in your diet first, slowly progressing towards a completely wholefood diet which includes a daily salad of fresh fruit and vegetables. You can start your supplements as soon as you like. But it might be a good plan to take just the multivitamin and mineral preparations for the first month, so that your system gets used to all the extra care you are lavishing on it.

If you go from a junk food diet without supplements to a wholefood one supplemented with a multiplicity of additional nutrients, your digestive system may well complain at the extreme contrast. Indigestion, nausea or constipation/diarrhoea will then convince you that the supplements do not agree with you, and you will cease to take them forthwith.

My advice is to add the supplements item by item over a period of three or four months, always remembering that, unlike drugs, vitamins and minerals take a comparatively long time to produce a noticeable effect.

Exercise

Similar advice is applicable to taking up exercise. Whatever type of exercise you decide to take up – if you have not exercised for years, do not be tempted to go on for too long. The first few deep breaths you take of fresh air often make you feel buoyant, and the stimulation of jogging, cycling or swimming (the excitement of actually having started!) can tempt you to continue for longer than is wise.

Keep to the times suggested in Table 2, Chapter Four, even if these do appear very short when reading through them. And *always* limber up first. In this way you will avoid painful pulled calf muscles.

Relaxation and Sex

Relaxation techniques *are* something you can start looking at seriously right from the start, with a view to learning and practising daily. Stress is likely to be your biggest enemy, and a daily yoga session, or half an hour spent in autohypnosis will help you to remain calm and cheerful while you slowly integrate your new plans into the rest of your life.

Regarding love-making, I do not need to say that the sooner you make some move to improve a less than perfect sexual relationship, the easier and better it will be for both of you. If you just cannot bring yourself to broach the subject, try suggesting to your husband or lover that he join you in a relaxation session. This may not appeal to him but at least he will ask you why *you* are keen on them. This can be your cue for letting him know that you want to improve many aspects of your lives, and that you feel a calmer and better tempered 'you' would go a long way to achieving that. You could then say casually: 'perhaps we'll get round to making love again soon/sharing our fantasies/reading a sexy book together' – whatever you have in mind! He may look askance but it will start him thinking!

I have referred many times in this book to 'you', and 'your life', as though your nearest and dearest, and other family members, were no more than shadowy figures on the periphery of your existence. The truth is, of course, that if you have a family, husband, children and parents are central to it, and you are very probably used, from long-established habit, to considering their interests before your own.

As I expect you have realized by now, all the lifestyle changes I have suggested will benefit your husband (and children if they are still at home) just as much as they will you. A change of diet can only improve their vitality and well-being, however healthy they may currently seem to be. Exercise is enormous fun if carried out in a family group – and if you *should* feel self-conscious jogging (there is no need to), there is safety in numbers!

Those around you will even benefit from your relaxation

sessions! They may well be sufficiently interested to take it up too – but even if they do not, you will be, in a short time, so much calmer and better tempered that they will regard the changes you have made as very much for the better. They may not be interested in supplements, but try to persuade them to take at least a natural multivitamin and chelated mineral supplement every day.

You may well find, though, that anyone anticipating a possible hangover will be sneaking half a dozen of your Efamol capsules; and that slimmers will be after your amino acid supplements for weight reduction!

A further element upon which will depend your success in making the menopause a change for the better is the cultivation of a positive mental attitude. This is sufficiently vital for me to say that, whatever your efforts in other directions, your life will certainly not change for the better without it. And that if you retain a really negative frame of mind for months on end, your life can only change for the worse.

This is in no sense a moral issue. There is nothing wicked in brooding over past grievances, moaning constantly about trivial problems, or despairing over present problems rather than deciding what to do about them. The only harm that comes of persistent negativity is to yourself, for it saps what is left of your energy and vitality, aggravates symptoms of all kinds and makes friends instinctively avoid your company.

A positive mental attitude is vital to health. Misery – including the type that is largely self-inflicted – is a stress factor many therapists and doctors believe is instrumental in causing physical changes which predispose us to disease. Anger, grief and chronic anxiety all play their part in depleting the strength of our immune defence mechanism, making us prey to infections, allergic responses, digestive upsets, muscular and skeletal disorders, and – it is now believed – to the abnormal cellular changes predisposing to cancer.

If you have had a negative attitude for so long now that you don't know how to change, alter one thing at a time. Start by *knowing* that your new wholefood diet will do you a great deal of good – and take pleasure in your meals, savouring the new textures, colours and flavours you will experience.

Pick a form of exercise you have always wanted to try – or take up something you used to do and abandoned. Choose something you actually like instead of martyring yourself in the cause of 'good health' – no good ever came out of doing it that way. Buy an attractive track suit (or swimming costume, or leotard and tights), and look forward to your workouts. And congratulate yourself on your achievement each time you complete your exercise routine.

Again, if you *are* a deeply negative person, book an appointment with a psychotherapist or hypnotherapist and talk about yourself and your problems. A sympathetic audience will make you feel much better quite quickly, and you will probably be encouraged to practise relaxation between therapy sessions.

The one thing you must avoid at all costs is dwelling on the past, either because it seems more attractive than the present and future, or because you 'cannot forget' past injuries you have suffered. You can forget the past well enough if you determine to cast it on one side and busy yourself with improving the present.

Some of the improvements you can think of may seem daunting. But *now* is the time to carry out the changes you've always wished for, and you are the person who is going to have to initiate them.

Firstly, think again about what I said about marriage in the chapter on sex and the menopause. If you are unhappy, make the effort to sit down and discuss the problems. If you haven't spoken for months – assess the situation and have a final try anyway. If that doesn't work out, then see a marriage guidance counsellor alone.

Easier divorce was not intended to make people give up on marriage rather than work to put it right. But at least it means that you do not have to live in misery – for the sake of the children or anyone else.

The same advice applies to your job, if you have one. If it is casual work to bring in a few pounds, and you feel indifferent to it, carry on with it for as long as you need the cash. But if you loathe your work and absolutely dread going there every day, do review the situation to see whether there is a way out.

Even if the alternative is applying for other jobs you do not think you would get, at least make the effort – and if you can do without the money, choose peace of mind and contentment in preference to spending hours every week doing something you dislike.

Shirley Conran says in her book *Superwoman* – 'Life is too short to stuff a mushroom.' I disagree about mushroom stuffing – but her principle is of course absolutely true. Don't waste time on fiddly jobs that don't deserve it – and don't waste precious hours of your life being wretched.

Take up a new hobby – there are plenty of free ones, such as learning about art from library books and visiting art galleries, or reading about music and listening to it on the radio. You can even go skuba diving, take your advanced drivers' test or learn to dance on ice.

Whatever you choose – *make sure you enjoy yourself!*

References

1 Padwick, M. and Whitehead, M., 'Oestrogen deficiency: causes, consequences and management', *Update*, August 15, 1985.

2 Sturdee, D. W., 'Which borderline menopausal symptoms respond to HRT?', *Modern Medicine*, November 1981.

3 Aitken, J. M., *BMJ*, Nov 10, 1984, 289, 1311.

4 Chaitow, Leon, 'Menopause', *Here's Health*, November 1983.

5 Campbell, S. and Whitehead, M. I., *Clinics in Obstetrics and Gynaecology*, 4, no. 1, *The Menopause* (Philadelphia: W. B. Saunders, 1977), pp. 31–47.

6 Osborn, M., *British Journal of Hospital Medicine*, 1984, 32, 126.

7 Vessey, M., *BMJ*, 1980, 281, 181.

8 Fowler, A., *BMJ*, 1983, 287, 286.

9 Goldman, L., 'Post-menopausal osteoporosis – a differing view', *Geriatric Medicine*, March 1984.

10 Whitehead, M. I., King, R. J. B., McQueen, J. and Campbell, S., 'Endometrial histology and biochemistry in climacteric women during oestrogen and oestrogen/progestogen therapy', *J R Soc. Med.*, 1979, 72, 322–7.

11 Knab, D. R., 'Oestrogen and endometrial carcinoma', *Obstetr. Gynaecol. Surv.*, 1977, 3, 267–81.

12 Studd, J. W. W. and Thom, M. H., *Progress in Obstetrics and Gynaecology* (Edinburgh: Churchill Livingstone, 1981), vol. 1, pp. 182–198.

13 *Here's Health*, December 1984.

14 Lust, J. B., *Raw Juice Therapy* (Thorsons Publishers Ltd, 1959).

15 Bricklin, Mark, *The Practical Encyclopedia of Natural Healing* (Rodale Press Inc., 1976), p. 171.

16 *New Health*, November 1983, p. 104.

17 Cannon, G., *New Health*, June 1985, p. 43.

18 Norfolk, D., *Fit For Life* (Hamlyn Books, 1981), p. 82.

19 Gardner, T., 'Yoga Therapy' in *The Practical Encyclopedia of Natural Healing*, ed. Mark Bricklin (Rodale Press Inc., 1976), p. 537.

20 Passwater, Richard A., *EPA – Marine Lipids* (Frelmore Ltd Health Publications, 1982).

21 *JAMA*, April 1983, 22/29, 249, 16, 2195.

22 *Medical News*, May 12, 1983.

23 Kenton, Leslie and Susannah, *Raw Energy* (Century, 1984).

24 Messegué, M., *Health Secrets of Plants and Herbs* (Pan Books, 1981), p. 131.

25 Lewith, G. T., *Acupuncture – Its Place in Western Medical Science* (Thorsons Publishers Ltd, 1982), p. 63.

26 Mann, Felix, *Acupuncture – Cure of Many Diseases* (Pan Books, 1973), p. 98.

27 Inglis, B. and West, R., *The Alternative Health Guide* (Michael Joseph, 1983), p. 112.

28 Kaye, Anna and Matchan, Don C., *Reflexology. Techniques of Foot Massage for Health and Fitness* (Thorsons Publishers Ltd, 1978), p. 19.

29 Inglis, B. and West, R., p. 115.

30 Brown, Sarah, *Vegetarian Kitchen* (British Broadcasting Corporation, 1984).

Index